Contemporary Issues *in* Animal and Veterinary Sciences

Dhirendra Kumar

Dibyendu Chakraborty

Pranav Kumar

Vikas Mahajan

SSPH

SATISH SERIAL PUBLISHING HOUSE

403, Express Tower, Commercial Complex
Azadpur, Delhi-110033 (India)
Phone : 011-27672852, Fax : 91-11-27672046
e-mail : info@satishserial.com, hkjain1975@yahoo.com
Website : www.satishserial.com

Published by :

SATISH SERIAL PUBLISHING HOUSE
403, Express Tower, Commercial Complex, Azadpur, Delhi-110033 (INDIA)
Phone : 011-27672852 Fax : 91-11-27672046
E-mail : info@satishserial.com, hkjain1975@yahoo.com

ISBN 978-93-88020-01-5

Composed, Designed & Printed in India

About the Authors

Dr. Dhirendra Kumar is presently working as Assistant Professor of Animal Genetics & Breeding at Sher-e-Kashmir University of Agricultural Sciences and Technology of Jammu (SKUAST-J), R.S.Pura, Jammu (J&K). Dr. Dhirendra is a recipient of Best Ph.D Thesis award,Appreciation Award (2),Distinguished Scientist Award, Excellence in Teaching Award, Young Scientist Award (2) and Life Science Leadership Award. He has also served as Organizing Secretary of International Conference (1), Joint Organizing Secretary of International Conference (1) and Co-Organizing Secretary of National Conference/Symposium (2) Presently he is the Principal Investigator of Network Project of NBAGR-ICAR on Characterization of Poonchi Chicken. He also acted as a Co-Principal Investigator under Network Projects of ICAR on "Characterization of Sheep and Goat". He was the co-project leader of the project "Capacity building/Training of Women Self Help Group members from Umeed as Community Paravets". He has published more than 40 research and review articles in reputed national and international scientific journals. He has edited three books. He has also contributed in scientific fields by means of popular articles, conference proceeding papers, short communications, chapters in books, manuals, edited publications, etc.

Dr. Dibyendu Chakraborty is presently working as Assistant Professor of Animal Genetics & Breeding at Sher-e-Kashmir University of Agricultural Sciences and Technology of Jammu (SKUAST-J), R.S.Pura, Jammu (J&K). Dr. Chakraborty, is a recipient of Excellence in Scientific Writing Award of the Society for Bioinformatics and Biological Sciences, Allahabad for the year of 2015. He is also awarded with Appreciation Awards by different scientific societies for his excellent contribution in the scientific fields. He has also served as Co-Organizing Secretary of one International and one National Symposiums. He was associated with two research project on "Characterization of Sheep and Goat" as a Co-Principal Investigator under Network Projects of ICAR. He has published more than 50 research and review articles in reputed national and international scientific journals. He has also contributed in scientific fields by means of popular articles, conference proceeding papers, short communications, chapters in books, manuals, edited publications and radio talk. He is also reviewer of different National and International Journals. His major contributions are in the field of Animal Breeding and Molecular Genetics.

Dr. Pranav Kumar is presently working as Assistant Professor (SS) in the Division of Veterinary & A.H. Extension at Faculty of Veterinary Sciences, R.S.Pura, SKUAST- Jammu. He has over 12 years of work experience. He has graduated from College of Veterinary Sciences, Hyderabad in 2001 and completed Master Degree in Veterinary Extension from IVRI, Izzatnagar, Bareilly. He has published 20 research papers and 02 review papers in NAAS rated journals. He has authored 11 book chapters, 21 popular articles, 4 case studies, 7 field manuals and few technical articles. He has co-authored a Textbook on "Livestock Entrepreneurship Management" published by NIPA, New Delhi. He received Young Scientist Award, Excellence in Teaching Award and Excellence in Extension Award for his contribution to teaching, research and extension in the field of Veterinary Extension from the reputed Extension Education Society. He has also served as Co-Organizing Secretary of one International Conference and core member committee of one National Conference. He was associated with two externally funded research projects as Co-PI funded by National Innovation Foundation (DST) & J&K State Rural Livelihoods Mission (JKSLRM) and presently associated with one on-going project funded by DST related to establishment of Women Technology Park in Jammu. He is also a reviewer of different NAAS rated Journals. His major contributions are in the field of documentation of indigenous technical knowledge related to low cost treatment of animal ailments, livestock entrepreneurship, organic dairy farming and development of dynamic web module for Scientific Dairy Practices and Broiler farming.

Dr. Vikas Mahajan is presently working as Assistant Professor (PhD in Animal Genetics & Breeding), Division of Instructional; Livestock Farm Complex, Faculty of Veterinary Sciences and Animal Husbandry, Sher-e-Kashmir University of Agricultural Sciences and Technology of Jammu (SKUAST-J), R.S.Pura, Jammu (J&K). Professional experience more than three years with a wide variety of publication, which includes research papers (23), books (05), Manual (02). He has edited two books. He has also contributed in scientific fields by means of popular articles, conference proceeding papers, short communications, chapters in books, manuals, edited publications, etc. He is also reviewer of different National and International Journals.

Preface

Veterinary science has benefited significantly from technological advances over recent years. The advances have contributed to faster animal health, production and reproduction improvement and more accurate diagnoses, and better treatments. Recent trends toward different reproductive and molecular techniques including sexing of semen, in-vitro maturation of oocytes, genetic screening for dieseases, genome editing, drug designing, next generation sequencing, animal products improvization helps to improve the productivity of animals.

With the advancement of clinical science now-a-days, a lot of options have innovated for management of different type of clinical cases. It is already possible to determine genotypes for pharmacogenomics-related with the advancement of new technologies in veterinary sciences. NGS helps to determine the order of bases as ingene-expression studies which can identify and quantify rare transcripts without having prior knowledge of a particular gene and also provide information regarding alternative splicing and sequence variation in identified genes. Such procedures would allow veterinarians to modify gene/gene combinations in animals to treat a range of different maladies and enhancing production. The advances in knowledge transfer technology to farmers at grassroot level also enhancing to adopt of new technologies and techniques among rural masses for sustainable development of animal productivity.

The chapters are invited from various researchers and academicians over the country. We are highly thankful to all the resource persons for their valuable contribution in this book.

The views expressed in this book are solemnly those of the authors. Despite the careful efforts have been in compilation of the present publication, if have been any errors may kindly be pardoned and brought to the notice for further improvement. We hope this present publication will be useful to students and academicians working in the field of Veterinary Sciences.

Happy Reading

Editors

Contents

Chapter 1

Use of Biomaterials in Veterinary Clinical Setup

D. K. DWIVEDI[1] AND A. K. GUPTA[2]

Division of Veterinary Surgery and Radiology
F.V.Sc & A.H, R.S.Pura, SKUAST-J, Jammu

With the advancement of clinical science now-a-days, we have lot of options for management of different type of clinical cases. One among them is the application of biomaterials for the management of damaged or compromised tissues/organs/system of body. These biomaterials not only helps in tissue regeneration but at the same time it also helps or augments or assists in normal functioning of the compromised tissues or organs or body system.

Any non-living material that can be used in biological system without exciting the immune system is known as biomaterial. Few important definitions are as follows: A biomaterial is a non-viable material used in a medical device, intended to interact with biological systems (Williams, 1987). Another definition is "Any material of natural or of synthetic origin that comes in contact with tissue, blood or biological fluids and intended for use in prosthetic, diagnostic, therapeutic or storage application" (Boretos and Eden,1984). The latest definition of Biomaterials are defined as "active substances capable of interaction with the surrounding tissues, without causing an immune response". The ability to augment the tissue regeneration and function as a part or whole of the organ has improved the scope of human as well as animal life. A variety of materials like sutures, needles, catheters, plates, tooth fillings are also very commonly used now a days in clinical practice (Zhu *et al., 2007*). Further, the availability of human/animal organs is difficult which has paved the way for the use of synthetic materials. Now-a-days, this has emerged into a separate branch of science known as biomaterial science, which deals with the biomaterials.

History

More than 2000 years ago, Romans, Chinese, and Aztec used gold in dentistry. Turn of last century, synthetic implants become available. In 1937, Poly methylmethacrylate (PMMA) was introduced in dentistry 1958, Rob suggests Dacron Fabrics can be used to fabricate an arterial prosthetic. In 1960, Charnley, used PMMA, ultrahigh-molecular-weight polyethylene and stainless steel for total hip replacement .Late 1960–early 1970's biomaterial field solidified and in 1975, Society for Biomaterials was formed.

Properties of Biomaterials

The requirements of biomaterials can be physical and biological. The physical requirements are highly important for the orthopaedic implants besides its biological requirements. The general requirements of biomaterials are as under:

i) Inert or specifically interactive
ii) Biocompatible
iii) Mechanically and chemically stable
iv) Biodegradable
v) Processable (for manufacturability)
vi) Non-thrombogenic (if blood-contacting)
vii) Sterilizable

Biocompatible (B)

Researchers have coined the word biomaterial and biocompatibility to indicate the biological performance of materials. Materials that are biocompatible are called biomaterials and the biocompatibility is descriptive term which indicates the ability of a material to perform with an appropriate host response in specific application. It is a general term meaning that a biomaterial, device or construct can be brought into direct contact with living tissue without:

a) Causing a harmful tissue reaction (pain, swelling or necrosis) that could compromise function.
b) Causing a systemic toxic reaction.
c) Having tumorigenic/Carcinogenic potential/Teratogenic

$B = f(X_1, X_2 ...... Xn)$

Where X : material, design, application, etc.

Biocompatibility testing includes procedures designed to evaluate

i) Cytotoxicity

ii) Acute, sub-chronic, and chronic toxicity

iii) Irritation to skin, eyes, and mucosal surfaces

iv) Sensitization

v) Hemocompatibility

vi) Short-term implantation effects

vii) Genotoxicity

Carcinogenicity and effects on reproduction, including developmental effects. These tests are performed on various laboratory animals and after getting appropriate results the materials is gradually shifted for its use in clinical cases.

Physical or mechanical properties of biomaterials or implants (Saini *et al.*, 2015)

a) Modulus of elasticity : Implant material with modulus of elasticity comparable to bone (18GPa) must be selected to ensure more uniform distribution of stress at implant and to minimize the relative movement at implant bone interface.

b) Tensile, compressive and shear strength: Implant material should have high tensile and compressive strength to prevent fracture and improve functional stability.

c) Yield strength, fatigue strength: An implant material should have high yield strength and fatigue strength to prevent brittle fracture under cyclic loading.

d) Ductility : Ductility in implant is necessary for contouring and shapping of an implant.

e) Hardness and toughness: Increase in hardness decreases the incidence of wear of implant material and increase in toughness prevents fracture of implants.

The biomaterial selected for its application must have appropriate level of mechanical and biological properties for getting successful result.

Surface Properties

a) Surface tension and surface energy : It determines the wettability of implant by wetting fluid (blood) and cleanliness of implant surface. Osteoblasts show improved adhesion on implant surface. Surface energy also affects adsorption of proteins.

b) Surface roughness : It influences the response of cells and tissue by increasing the surface area of the implant adjacent to bone and thereby improving the cell attachment to bone.

Classification of Biomaterials

A variety of biomaterials are presently employed in medicine and these biomaterials are classified on the basis of different criteria like source of material, its activity within the biological system, chemical property of biomaterials, etc. Some important classes of biomaterials are as under:

General classes of biomaterials (Hawal, 1998):

a) Class I-Materials do not directly contact body tissue

b) Class II-Contact body tissue intermittently or instantly

c) Class III-Constantly contacting body tissues: It is further divided into Bioinert, Bioactive and Biodegradable, etc.

On the basis of origin of material we may classify as:

A. Natural / Biologically Derived

a) Proteins, Polysaccharides

b) Acellular diaphragm: Used for wound repair, herniorraphy, etc.

c) Acellular pericardium: Used for wound repair, herniorraphy, etc.

d) Amniotic membrane: Used in wound repair, Corneal ulcers treatment, etc

e) Collagen, Chitosin, Alginate, Pectin: Used in wound management

B. Synthetic / Materials Synthesized in Laboratories (PMMA, PVC, etc.)

a) Metals (Fe, Cr, Co, Ni, Ti, Mo, W, etc.)
b) Polymers (PVC, PMMA, Polyamide, etc.)
c) Ceramics (Alumina, Zirconia, HA, TCP, etc.)
d) Biocomposite

On the basis of activity of material in biological environment, we may classify into (Cao and Hench, 1996; Hench, 1998; Shin *et al.*, 2003):

a) Bioinert (Minimal interaction within biological system) ex: Zirconia ($Zr\ O_2$), Alumina ($Al\ 2O_3$), UHMW-PE, etc.
b) Bioactive: Interacts with biological system ex: Synthetic HA, Bioglass, etc.
c) Bioresorbable/Biodegradable: Starts to dissolve within body and slowly replace by advancing tissue ex: Tricalcium phosphate (TCP), etc.

Blood derived biomaterials (Burnouf *et al.*, 2013).

The basis for development of biomaterial is blood coagulation.

a) Fibrin sealant: Haemostasis ,used in cardiac, liver and spleen surgery.
b) Platelet gel: Wound repair and tissue regeneration.
c) Platelet fibrin glue: Wound repair.
d) Platelet rich fibrin: Wound repair.

Metallic Implant Materials

Metals have been used almost exclusively for load bearing implants, such as hip and knee prostheses and fracture fixation wires, pins, screws and plates. Three material groups dominate biomedical metals: stainless steel, cobalt-chromium-molybdenum alloy and titanium and titanium alloys. The main considerations in selecting metals and alloys for biomedical applications are their excellent electrical and thermal conductivity, biocompatibility, appropriate mechanical properties, corrosion resistance and reasonable cost

(*Patel et al., 2012*). The various advantages and disadvantages of metallic implants are as under:

Advantages : Fatigue resistance, Wear resistance, Easy fabrication, Easy to sterilize, Shape memory, High strength.

Disadvantages : Corrosion, Metal ion sensitivity and toxicity, Metallic looking, High moduls.

Examples: Stainless steel (316L), Co-Cr alloys, Ti6Al4V, Au-Ag-Cu-Pd alloys, Amalgam (AgSnCuZnHg), Ni-Ti, Titanium, etc.

Polymeric Biomaterial

The development of polymeric biomaterials can be considered as an evolutionary process. Reports on the applications of natural polymers as biomaterials date back thousands of years. Polymers are most widely used materials in biomedical applications. Polymers are organic materials that form large chain made up of many repeating units. The uses of polymeric biomaterials are more diverse in comparison to metallic materials, but their interchange ability is not as great. In most applications the polymers have little or no competition with other type of materials. The major advantage and disadvantage of polymeric biomaterials are as under:

Advantages : Easy to make complicated items,Tailorable physical & mechanical properties,Surface modification,Immobilize cell, etc,Biodegradable,Light weight, Flexibility, Rsistant to biochemical attack.

Disadvantages : Leachable compounds,Absorb water & proteins, etc, Surface contamination,Wear & breakdown, Biodegradation difficult to sterilize.

A few major classes of polymers are as follows : PMMA (Polymethyl methacrylate), PVC (Polyvinyl chloride), PLA/PGA (Polylactic acid or Polyglactic acid), PE, PP (Polypropylene), PA (Polyamide), PTFE (Polytetrafluroethylene), PET, PUR, Silicones, etc.

Bioceramics

Creamics are nonorganic, nonmetallic, nonpolymer materials manufactured by compacting and sintering at elevated temperature. Ceramics are polycrystalline materials. The main characteristics of ceramics are hardness and brittleness, great strength and stiffness, resistance to corrosion and wear and low density. Ceramics are typically electrical and thermal insulators. Ceramics are used in several different fields, such as dentistry, orthopaedics and as medical sensors. The various advantages and disadvantages of ceramic biomaterials are as under:

Advantages : High compression strength, Wear & corrosion resistance, Can be highly polished, Bioactive/inert.

Disadvantages : High modulus (mismatched with bone), Low strength in tension, Low fracture toughness, Difficult to fabricate.

Selection of Biomaterial

The process of material selection should ideally be for a logical sequence involving:

a) Analysis of the problem

b) Consideration of requirement

c) Consideration of available material and their properties

d) Choice of material

e) Acceptable cost/benefit ratio.

Applications of Biomaterials with Reference to Veterinary Practice

Biomaterials are now used extensively in veterinary practice also but still veterinarians are far behind in comparison to human applications of biomaterials. The main reason behind this is the paucity of work on animals. But in human lot of research work was conducted. Further, cost is an important hindrance in application of these biomaterials in veterinary practice. Some common applications of biomaterials in veterinary practice are as under (*Blackford et al., 2006*):

Material	Implant form
Carbon	Fibres, implant coatings, orthopaedic rods, meshes
Ceramics	Orthopaedic devices, Bone lattice, implant coatings
CO-Cr	Prosthetic implants
Collagen	Suture material , haemostatic sponge
Cyanoacrylate	Tissue adhesives
Gelatin	Haemostatic sponge

Latex rubber	Surgical drain
Poliglecaprone, Polyamide, Polybuster,	Surgical sutures
Polydiaxanone	Surgical sutures, surgical staples, orthopaedic pins
Polyester	Surgical suture, surgical mesh, vascular graft
Polyethylene	Tubings, catheters, Joint implants
Polyglactin	Surgical sutures, surgical mesh, surgical staples
Polyglycolic acid	Surgical sutures, surgical mesh, surgical staples, orthopaedic implants
Polylactide	Orthopaedic implants
PMMA	Tissue cement ,Intra ocular lens
Polyoxymethylene	Orthopaedic washer
Polypropylene	Surgical sutures, surgical mesh
Polyurethrane	Pacemaker loeads, vascular grafts
PVC	Tubings, catheters
Silicone rubber	Tubings, pacemaker leads, intraocular prostheses
Silk	Surgical sutures
Stainless steel	Surgical suture , surgical mesh, surgical staples, IMP, Circlage wires, Plates etc
Small intestine sub-mucosa	Collagen scaffold for tissue regeneration
Surgical gut	Surgical sutures
Titanium/alloys	Bone plates, screws, prosthetic implants

Detoriation of Biomaterials

a) Corrossion
b) Degradation
c) Calcification
d) Mechanical loading
e) Combined

Success of a biomaterial or an implant depends on three (3) major factors (Manivasagam *et al.*, 2010)

a) The properties (mechanical, chemical and tribological) of biomaterial in question
b) Biocompatibility
c) Health condition of recipient
d) Competency of surgeon

References

1. Boretos, J.W. and Eden M. (1984). Contemporary biomaterials. Material and Host response. Clinical applications. New technology and legal aspects.Noyes publications. *Park ridge.NJ* pp. 232-233.
2. Blackford, J.T., Blackford, L.W., Disegi, J. and Bohner, M.(2006).Biomaterials, surgical implants and instruments. Equine surgery by Auer and stick, Elsevier Saunders,3rd edition, pp. 96-110.
3. Burnouf, T., Goubran, H. A., Chen, T. M., Ou, K. L., Ekiaby, M. E. and Radosevic M. (2013).Blood derived biomaterials and platelet growth factors in regenerative medicine. *Blood Rev.*, 27: 77-79.
4. Cao, W. and hench, L.L. (1996). Bioactive materials. *Ceram. Int.*, 8842: 493-507.
5. Hawal, S.(1998).Recent advances in Biomaterials. Yonsei Med. J., 39(2): 87-96.
6. Hench, L.L. (1998). Biomaterials: a forcast for future biomaterials, 19: 1419-1423.
7. Manivasagam, G., Dhinasekaran, D. and Rajamanikam, A. (2010). Biomedical implants: Corrosion and its prevention-A review. *Recent patents on corrosion scienece*, 2: 40-54.
8. Patel, N. R. and Gohil, P. P. A review of biomaterials. *Int. J. Emerg. Tech. Adv. Eng.*, Vol 2, April 2012.
9. Shin, H., Jo, S.and Mikos, A. G. (2003). Biomimetic materials for tissue engineering. *Biomaterials*, 24: 4353-4364.
10. Saini, M., Singh, Y., Arora, P., Arora, V. and Jain, K.(2015).Implant biomaterial :A comprehensive review. *World J.Clin. Cases*, 3(1): 52-57.
11. Williams, D.F. (1987). Definitions in Biomaterials. Proceedings of a consensus conference of European Society for Biomaterials, Chester, England, march 3-5, 1986, Vol 4 New York, Elsevier, 1420-1422.
12. Zhu, S. L.,Wang, X. M.,Qin, F. X. and Inoue, A. (2007). A new Ti-based bulk glassy alloy with potential for biomedical applications. *Material Sci. Eng.*, A (459): 233-237.

□□□

Chapter 2

Oocyte Development under Heat Stress Ordering a Fried Egg

JAFRIN ARA AHMED[1] AND NAWAB NASHIRUDDULLAH[2]

[1] Division of Veterinary Physiology & Biochemistry
[2] Division of Veterinary Pathology
Faculty of Veterinary Sciences & Animal Husbandry, Sher-e-Kashmir University of Agricultural University Sciences & Technology- Jammu, RS Pura-181102, Jammu & Kashmir, India

Introduction

Elevated ambient temperature is one of the major factors responsible for reduced fertility in farm animals (Ealy *et al.*, 1995). Heat stress can have profound effects on most aspects of reproductive function in both sexes of mammals. These include disruptions in spermatogenesis in the male and oocyte development, oocyte maturation, early embryonic development, foetal and placental growth and lactation (Hansen, 2009). Many of the harmful effects are a consequence of hyperthermia or a systemic compensatory effect by the body to counter it.

Events in Oocyte Maturation

The oocyte undergoes a remarkable array of developmental changes immediately before and just after fertilization. The events of oocyte maturation as reviewed by Barnes and Sirard (2000), is the intricate process by which the oocyte prepares at the nuclear, cytoplasmic, and molecular levels for fertilization by reductive division of the maternal DNA and dynamic changes in intracellular organization. Fully grown oocytes have an intact nucleus (or germinal vesicle, GV) and are maintained in prophase I arrest until they are recruited for ovulation. This arrest can last weeks to months in rodents, or months to decades in humans (Picton *et al.*, 1998) and is relieved in oocytes that are 'selected' for ovulation during each hormonal cycle upon a luteinizing hormone (LH) surge (Eppig *et al.*, 1996) or in culture, after removal from the follicular environment (Pincus and Enzmann, 1935).

The short time between the LH surge and ovulation (approximately 12–14 hrs) is referred to as meiotic maturation, when the oocyte progresses through the bulk of meiosis during this period. During meiotic maturation, the nuclear envelope breaks down (a process known as germinal vesicle breakdown), and the oocyte proceeds from meiosis I to meiosis II without an intervening interphase. The maturing oocyte also undergoes cytoplasmic modifications in preparation for early developmental events that occur upon fertilization, such as sperm nuclear decondensation (Perreault *et al.*, 1988) and calcium oscillations (Ajduk *et al.*, 2008). The end of meiotic maturation is marked by the establishment of a second meiotic arrest at metaphase II (Cooley, 1995), at which point this single cell is now called an egg.

Various developmental hallmark events mark the oocyte maturation process :

Nuclear maturation: This is to reduce the number of copies of maternal chromatin from and requires progression from prophase I of meiosis through metaphase I, anaphase I, telophase I and, re-arrest at metaphase II (MII) with extrusion of the first polar body containing two copies of DNA. The accumulation of maturation promoting factor (MPF) components, cyclin B1 and p34cdc2 kinase, is necessary for resumption of meiosis (Levesque and Sirard, 1996).

Cytoplasmic maturation: The majority of organelles migrate from the inner regions of the oocyte to a cortical position mediated by the cytoskeletal network (Hyttel *et al.*, 1997; Ferreira *et al.*, 2009). Mitochondria cluster near other organelles and nuclear material in association with increased ATP production as maturation progresses (Stojkovic *et al.*, 2001), and is necessary for protein synthesis during maturation (Krisher and Bavister, 1998).

Molecular maturation: Molecular maturation refers to the accumulation and storage of RNA and proteins during oocyte growth for use during and after meiotic maturation, often referred to as an accumulation of a legacy of the instructions accumulated during the GV-stage that controls both, the nuclear and the cytoplasmic progression (Sirard, 2001).

In vitro Embryonic Development

Since the birth of the first *in vitro* produced embryos, many attempts have been made to improve *in vitro* production (IVP) by refining maturation, fertilization, and culture conditions. However, the efficiency of the *in vitro* procedure to produce morulae and blastocysts remain lower than *in vivo* (Merton *et al.*, 2003). A number of factors influence the survival of embryos produced with *in vitro* systems. These include media composition (Thompson, 2000), oocyte quality (Blondin and Sirard, 1995), environment and embryo genotype. The developmental competence of oocytes produced by *in vitro* maturation (IVM) is far inferior to those undergoing maturation *in vivo*. It is thought that many of the essential biochemical pathways to complete oocyte maturation prior to fertilization are incomplete or inadequate during IVM of oocytes.

For the success of *in vitro* embryo production, several barriers need to be overcome. Optimizing the culture medium to produce an *in vitro* environment similar to the microenvironment in the oviduct and uterus (Yuan *et al.*, 2003) is an important step toward achieving this goal. Embryos of all mammalian species encounter a developmental block, when they are removed from their natural environment. In bovine, this developmental arrest takes place between the 8 and 16 cell stage (Thibault, 1966) and was first overcome through the use of co-culture systems involving oviduct epithelial cells (Eyestone *et al.*, 1991) or other cell lineage (Myers *et al.*, 1994) in standard tissue culture media (TCM199). The exact effective mechanism has not been determined, but presumably mediated through growth factors regulating embryo development or removal of toxic media components (Killian, 2004).

Newer culture media have been designed and optimised for embryo requirements without the need for co-culture. One of the first media designed for this purpose was synthetic oviduct fluid or SOF (Fukui *et al.*, 1991) established from the composition of bovine oviduct fluid. Recently, the use of sequential media have been proposed for varying requirements of the different evolutionary stages of the embryo (Gardner *et al.*, 2000); for example, a lesser incorporation of glucose in early cleaving embryos due to its toxicity, whereas more glucose in the medium during morula stage for further development (Donnay *et al.*, 2002; Gardner *et al.*, 2000).

Heat Stress

Heat stress can be defined as the sum of the environmental variables external to the bodily system of a homeothermic animal that acts to displace the body temperature from its resting state to conditions that are higher than the animal's thermoneutral zone (Lee, 1965). Elevated ambient temperature is one of the major factors responsible for reduced fertility in farm animals (Ealy *et al.*, 1995). The viability of cow oocytes and embryos is lower during the hot seasons than during the cooler seasons (Monty and Racowsky, 1987; Al-Katani *et al.*, 2002). A variety of factors have been attributed to this seasonal depression of reproductive performance, including-suboptimal environment, managerial changes, age, and species-specific sensitivity to those factors (Badinga *et al.*, 1985). High Effective Ambient Temperature (HEAT), a combination of high temperature with humidity changes an animal's physiological core temperature and is one of the major factors responsible for low reproductive performance in domestic animals during the hot seasons. The Temperature humidity index (THI) incorporates both ambient wet/dry bulb temperatures and relative humidity, and is universally used as a heat stress index for livestock production (Garcia-Ispierto *et al.*, 2006). The maximum THI (i.e. maximum temperature and minimum humidity) calculated for dairy cattle is 72 (Thom, 1959; Johnson *et al.*, 1962) and 68 for high producing dairy cattle (Finch, 1986; Zimbelman *et al.*, 2009) because of the added metabolism of milk production. Improving reproductive efficiency during periods of HEAT therefore, becomes a major challenge for animal producers in tropical and subtropical areas (Ju, 2005).

Hot environments can increase blood, rectal and uterine temperatures, suppress puberty (Kurowicka *et al.*, 2006); ovarian cyclicity (Christenson, 1980); ovulation (Rozenboim *et al.*, 2007); spermatogenesis, fertility (Kunavongkrit *et al.*, 2005); oogenesis and embryogenesis (Putney *et al.*, 1989; Edwards and Hansen, 1997; Beere, 2004; Lawrence *et al.*, 2004); and reduce conception and pregnancy rates (Christenson, 1980; Putney *et al.*, 1989) in different domestic animals.

Although heat induced cell damage and other deleterious effects on oocyte or embryo viability have been documented, yet the underlying mechanisms remain poorly understood (Ju, 2005).

Wrzal (2006), effectively summarised the effects of stress/heat shock response and include: i) inhibition of DNA synthesis, transcription, RNA processing and translation; ii) inhibition of progression through the cell cycle; iii) denaturation and misaggregation of proteins; iv) increased degradation of proteins through both proteosomal and lysosomal pathways; v) disruption of cytoskeletal components; vi) alterations in metabolism that lead to net reduction in cellular ATP; and vii) changes in membrane permeability that lead to an increase in intracellular Na^+, H^+ and Ca^{2+} (Lindquist, 1986; Sonna *et al.*, 2002; Jaattela, 1999).

In mammalian cells, non-lethal heat shock produces changes in gene expression and in the activity of expressed proteins in a stress/heat shock response (Sonna *et al.*, 2002; Parsell and Lindquist, 1993). This response characteristically includes an increase in thermo-tolerance, the ability to survive subsequent, more severe heat stresses, as well as cross-tolerance to other stressors (Creagh *et al.*, 2000). These characteristics of the stress/heat shock response earned it the well-known name of the chaperone system, which protects the cell from damage and in extreme stress situations leads to apoptosis and even necrosis (Ishikawa *et al.*, 1999). A large group of functionally related proteins have been found to be induced during heat stress (De Maio, 1999). These proteins are called Heat Shock Proteins (HSP) and their expressions have been found to be transcriptionally regulated. HSPs are molecular chaperones whose biological role is to maintain the unfolded, newly-synthesized proteins and allow them to traverse biological membranes or different cellular compartments such as the endoplasmic reticulum (ER) and mitochondria (Ju, 2005). Chaperones also prevent proteins from denaturing during and after stresses (Ang *et al.*, 1991).

Heat Stress and Oocyte Maturation

Heat stress cannot be studied *in vivo*, and therefore one has to resort to *in vitro* models that have the added advantage of isolating the indirect effects on the follicle or the endometrium. Generally, heat stress studies are conducted near visceral temperatures that are above those in the ovary. Determination of changes in ovum components is necessary as oocyte contributes more than 99 per cent of cytoplasm, and half the genetic material to the developing embryo (Schrock *et al.*, 2007).

The oocyte remains sensitive to heat stress through the period of oocyte maturation (Hansen, 2013). There are also direct effects of elevated temperature on nuclear maturation, spindle formation, cortical granule distribution, free radical formation, mitochondrial function (Payton *et al.*, 2004; Roth and Hansen, 2004, 2005; Ju *et al.*, 2005; Soto and Smith, 2009; Andreu-Vázquez *et al.*, 2010). Heat stress may also lead to apoptosis of the oocytes (Roth and Hansen, 2004) and also of the cumulus cells (Arav and Roth, 2008) that reduce their expansion and development competence.

In an excellent treatise on the consequences of heat stress in the female gamete, Maya-Soriano (2012) reviewed various effects encompassing ovarian follicles, steroidogenesis, oocytes, cumulus cells and embryos. The negative effects on the oocyte may include alterations in the cytoplasmic and nuclear maturation, protein expression, membrane alterations, induction of apoptosis, premature aging and overall developmental competence.

The pre-ovulatory stage is most sensitive to elevated temperature as has been observed in cattle (Ingraham *et al.*, 1976), pigs (Tseng, 2004) and sheep (Dutt, 1961). At the core temperature of 39°C, optimal cortical granular exocytosis, resumption of meiosis and pronuclear development occurs in bovines, which are otherwise considered temperature dependant (Sugiyama *et al.*, 2007). An increase in temperature interferes with oocyte maturation, subsequent fertilization and embryogenesis. These changes are hypothesized to be brought about by alterations in follicular fluid content (Wolfenson *et al.*, 1997), sustaining follicular cells (Shimizu *et al.*, 2005; Torres-Junior *et al.*, 2008), or even induced chromosomal errors (Tarin *et al.*, 1996). Whatever the underlying mechanism, heat stress does inhibit dominance of the principal follicle and the contained oocyte (Al-Katani *et al.*, 2002) and perhaps allow others of reduced competence to develop into embryo (Payton *et al.*, 2004; Roth and Hansen, 2004) often the leading cause of reduced fertility rates. The duration and severity of heat stress is the most important underlying factor governing the associated effects and ultimate fate of the oocyte/embryo.

In the phase of follicular growth, oocyte quality can be compromised by heat stress depending on temperature (Edwards and Hansen, 1996) or duration (Payton *et al.*, 2004) and may require about 2-3 subsequent oestrous cycles for recovery and generation of competent oocytes (Roth *et al.*, 2001).

Intracellular Events in Oocyte Maturation Induced by Heat Stress

Heat stress does take a major toll on the internal organelles of the oocyte, as has been reported during germinal vesicle stage (Payton *et al.*, 2004) or early stages of maturation (Edwards and Hansen, 1997; Roth and Hansen, 2004). Damage to the cytoskeleton by structural defects of microtubules and filaments (Tseng, 2004) including reorganization of the constituent actin filaments in mild temperature changes, resulting in collapse of intermediary actin and tubulin networks causing aggregation of vimentin and other filamentous proteins during severe temperature changes (Welch and Suhan, 1985; Toivola *et al.*, 2010); re-localization of organelles and breakdown of intracellular transport mechanisms of Golgi, endoplasmic reticulum, reduction of mitochondria and lysosomes numbers (Welch and Suhan, 1985); drop in ATP levels (Patriarca and Maresca, 1990), decrease in protein synthesis by 30-50 per cent (Edwards and Hansen, 1996; Edwards and Hansen, 1997), etc., all culminate to impose severe imbalance in the affected cells due to heat stress.

Nuclear Maturation : Heat shock induced around 40-41°C greatly reduce the number of oocytes reaching MII stage, being arrested in either of MI, AI or TI stages than their 38.5°C counterparts (Roth and Hansen, 2005). Heat stress causes an increase by 30% in inducing MI stage of nuclear maturation amongst heat-stress matured COCs and decreases the metaphase II stage by approximately 75% (Ahmed *et al.*, 2016). The meiotic spindle is particularly susceptible to temperature changes (Aman and Parks, 1994). The altered or elongated meiotic spindle is the predominant change occurring in the oocytes causing the reduction of microtubules or their aberrant formation (Ju *et al.*, 2005) and disorganization of chromosomal alignment (Roth and Hansen, 2005). Defects may reflect in the altered chromosome separation during fertilization and subsequent embryonic division (Streffer, 1984) or ultimately chromosomal imbalance and cell death (Ju *et al.*, 2005).

Cytoplasmic Maturation : Being less tolerant to thermal stress, changes in the cytoplasm are more pronounced than those of the nucleus (Wang *et al.*, 2008). The salient feature of cytoplasmic maturation after resumption of meiosis is the migration of cortical granules from Golgi with the help of actin microfilaments, through the oolema to the vitelline surface below the plasma membrane. Heat stress may cause either an incomplete migration due to structural and organizational loss of microfilaments (Ju and Tseng, 2004; Rivera *et al.*, 2004), or a pre-mature translocation of cortical granules possibly due to induced premature aging of oocytes (Lawrence *et al.*, 2004; Edwards *et al.*, 2005; Schrock *et al.*, 2007). Besides, microtubular alterations are also attributed to improper translocation of mitochondria around the meiotic spindle (Ju and Tseng, 2004; Ju, 2005; Roth and Hansen, 2005), compounded by a loss of mitochondrial membrane potential (Soto and Smith, 2009) that are otherwise vital for normal metabolism during the maturation process.

Induction of Apoptosis : The mechanism by which heat stress leads to a disruption in developmental competence of the oocyte remains unclear; however, one of the processes that may be involved is apoptosis, although there have been few studies on extrinsic or intrinsic control systems in reproduction for its activation (Roth and Hansen, 2004). Heat shock, for example, induces apoptosis in many cell types (Boreham *et al.*, 1997; Mosser *et al.*, 1997; Fuse *et al.*, 1998). Later, Paula-Lopes and Hansen (2002a) not only provided indication that heat shock, which is a cellular stress, can induce apoptosis in pre-implantation embryos, but also suggested that it was a developmentally regulated phenomenon. The effect of physiologically relevant elevated temperatures (41°C) induced on *in vitro* matured bovine oocytes were found to have a profound influence on its development competence with resulting pathological effects including ultrastructural changes, induction of apoptosis and expression of various pro- and anti-apoptotic protein markers (Ahmed, 2014; Ahmed *et al.*, 2017). The patterns of heat shock induced caspase activity were remarkably parallel to apoptosis. In another study, Paula-Lopes and Hansen (2002b) suggested that exposure to a mild heat shock could be a means of providing thermo tolerance that can protect embryos from heat-induced apoptosis. Tseng *et al.* (2006) also opined that there may be a link between apoptosis and heat shock as it compromised the developmental competence of matured porcine oocytes, although not closely associated with the expression of oocyte hsp70.

Studies by Soto and Smith (2009) provided evidence that heat shock induced apoptosis in bovine oocytes involves Bax and BH4 domain-dependent pathways. They have also documented that caspase-9 and -3/7 activity are critical effectors of heat shock induced apoptosis in oocytes exposed to caspase-9 inhibitor (z-LEHDfmk), as they demonstrated decreased DNA fragmentation detected by TUNEL labelling and increased proportion of oocytes that became blastocysts after insemination; strongly indicating the involvement of the mitochondrial intrinsic pathway in this process. These evidences suggest mitochondrial dysfunction as one probable factor that determine the magnitude of negative effects of stresses on oocyte developmental competence and apoptosis, as mitochondria play an important role in the integration and transmission of cell death signals mediated by the Bcl-2 family proteins (Soto and Smith, 2009). In an experiment on bovine oocytes, Nabenishi *et al.* (2012) found that 1 μM cyclosporine A (an inhibitor of mitochondrial permeability transition pore opening) treatment before IVM may mitigate reduced mitochondrial activity, decrease number of apoptotic cumulus cells under heat shock, and improve the nuclear maturation and developmental competence.

Apoptosis have also been found to be activated by the sphingomyelin pathway, generating the second messenger ceramide (Mathias *et al.*, 1998) which regulate the subsequent signalling cascade through Bcl-2, Apaf-1 and caspases. The fact that only a fraction of oocytes experience apoptosis when exposed to heat stress, points out to a possibility that some oocytes are better equipped to survive stress (Maya-Soriano, 2012) because they differ in the amounts of protective heat shock proteins like HSP70,though limited in its production (Edwards and Hansen, 1996; Edwards *et al.*, 1997).

Aging : The fertile lifespan of the oocytes may be greatly reduced under heat stress with the advent of premature aging and alteration of maturation kinetics (Payton *et al.*, 2003; Edwards *et al.*, 2005) invariably reducing its developmental competence (Fissore *et al.*, 2002). The cortical granular exocytosis occurred prematuredly prior to fertilization which is responsible for enlargement of the perivitelline space and altered zonapellucida properties (Okada *et al.*, 1993).

Membrane Alterations : Heat stress has also been associated with alterations in the phospholipid composition (Zeron *et al.*, 2001) as a result of peroxidative injury (Takahashi *et al.*, 2003) causing an altered protein: lipid ratio that increases the fluidity of the membrane (Vigh *et al.*, 2007) and affects the structure of the zonapellucida and microvilli pattern (Ju *et al.*, 1999). The resultant effect is an increase in membrane permeability accompanied consequently by altered ionic homeostasis and a decrease in cytosolic pH (Piper *et al.*, 2003).

Effect of Heat Stress on Cumulus Cells

The central role of the cumulus cells is to nurture the oocyte during maturation up to the MII stage (Tanghe *et al.*, 2002) through gap junctions (Moor *et al.*, 1980) that facilitates exchange of nutrient and chemical signals (Warnes *et al.*, 1977). Around meiotic resumption the cumulus cells withdraw from the oocyte with increasing production of hyaluronic acid (Chen *et al.*, 1990). During oxidative stress they protect the oocyte with increased glutathione content (Tatemoto *et al.*, 2000).

Heat stress may affect cumulus cells that indirectly influence ovum development or fertilization ability (Zhang *et al.*, 1995). Heat stress significantly reduces cumulus expansion by approximately 20% and decreases the expansion of grade A and B grade COC diameters by approximately 50% and 40%, respectively (Ahmed *et al.*, 2016). Sustained exposure to heat stress has been reported to reduce the hyaluronic acid production and cumulus cell expansion (Lenz *et al.*, 1983) while increasing DNA damage (Yuan *et al.*, 2008).

Conclusion

Elevated ambient temperature is associated with reduced fertility in animals. Associated with many systemic effects, it has a profound negative influence on the reproductive system including the maturation and fertilization of the oocytes. It is evident from *in vitro* studies that heat stress is deleterious to oocyte competence and viability. Since many of the heat stress studies on oocytes are under *in vitro* conditions, speculative presumptions can be made over similar negative effects in oocytes under *in vivo* conditions as well. In the present scenario of global warming, heat stress due to elevated temperatures has a significant relevance. Planet earth has seen drastic changes over recent years most of which have been blamed on anthropic factors. The concerns of global warming trends have been in the limelight especially in the face of predictions that the average surface temperature have risen about 0.6°C through the 20th century. With the increasing temperature changes there is a speculation that reproductive failures and infertility may increase. Although the body has tremendous potential to cope with changing environs and compensate for changes, yet it does take a toll on the bodily systems. It is, therefore, pertinent that measures are adopted through adequate intervention strategies so the deleterious effects are appropriately countered and the processes of life and its propagation restored.

References

1. Ahmed, J.A. (2014). Antioxidant Intervention during *in vitro* Maturation-Fertilization and Expression of Certain Apoptotic Genes in Heat Stress Induced Bovine Oocytes. PhD thesis. Assam Agricultural University, Guwahati, India.
2. Ahmed, J.A.; Nashiruddullah, N.; Dutta, D.; Biswas, R.K. and Borah, P. (2017). Cumulus cell expansion and ultrastructural changes in *in vitro* matured bovine oocytes under heat stress. *Iranian J. Vet. Res.*, 18: 203-207.
3. Ahmed, J.A.; Dutta, D.J. and Nashiruddullah, N. (2016). Comparative efficacy of antioxidant retinol, melatonin, and zinc during *in vitro* maturation of bovine oocytes under induced heat stress. *Turk. J. Vet. Anim. Sci.*, **4**: 365-373.
4. Ajduk, A.; Malagocki, A. and Maleszewski, M. (2008). Cytoplasmic maturation of mammalian oocytes: development of a mechanism responsible for sperm-induced Ca2+ oscillations. *Reprod. Biol.*, **8**: 3–22.
5. Al-Katani, Y.M.; Paula-Lopes, F.F. and Hansen, P.J. (2002). Effect of season and exposure to heat stress on oocyte competence in Holstein cows. *J. Dairy Sci.*, **85**: 390-396.
6. Aman, R.R. and Parks, J.E. (1994). Effects of cooling and rewarming on the meiotic spindle and chromosomes of *in vitro*-matured bovine oocytes. *Biol. Reprod.*, **50**(1): 103-110.
7. Andreu-Vázquez, C.; López-Gatius, F.; García-Ispierto, I.; Maya-Soriano, M.J.; Hunter, R.H. and López-Béjar, M. (2010). Does heat stress provoke the loss of a continuous layer of cortical granules beneath the plasma membrane during oocyte maturation? *Zygote*, **18**: 293-299.
8. Ang, D.; Liberek, K.; Skowyra, D.; Zylicz, M. and Georgopoulos, C. (1991). Biological role and regulation of the universally conserved heat shock proteins. *J. Biol. Chem.*, **266**: 24233-24236.
9. Arav, A. and Roth, Z. (2008). Do chilling injury and heat stress share the same mechanism of injury in oocytes? *Mol. Cell. Endrocrinol.*, **282**: 150-152.
10. Badinga, L.; Collier, R.J.; Thatcher, W.W. and Wilcox, C.J. (1985). Effects of climatic and management factors on conception rate of dairy cattle in subtropical environment. *J. Dairy Sci.*, **68**: 78-85.
11. Barnes, F.L. and Sirard, M.A. (2000). Oocyte maturation. *Seminars Reprod. Med.*, **18**: 123-131.
12. Beere, H.M. (2004). The stress of dying: the role of heat shock proteins in the regulation of apoptosis. *J. Cell Sci.*, **117**: 2641-2651.
13. Blondin, P. and Sirard, M.A. (1995).Oocyte and follicular morphology as determining characteristics for developmental competence in bovine oocytes. *Mol. Reprod. Develop.*, **41**(1): 54-62.

14. Boreham, D.R.; Doling, J.A.; Maves, S.R.; Miller, S.; Morrison, D.P. and Mitchel, R.E.J. (1997). Heat-induced thermal tolerance and radiation resistance to apoptosis in human lymphocytes. *Biochem. Cell Biol.*, **75**: 393–397.

15. Chen, L.; Wert, S.E.; Hendrix, E.M.; Russell, P.T.; Cannon, M. and Larsen, W.J. (1990). Hyaluronic acid synthesis and gap junction endocytosis are necessary for normal expansion of cumulus mass. *Mol. Reprod.Develop.*, **26**: 236-247.

16. Christenson, R.K. (1980). Environmental influences on the postpartum animal. *J. Anim. Sci.*, **51**: 53-67.

17. Cooley, L. (1995). Oogenesis: variations on a theme. *Develop. Genet.*, **16**: 1–5.

18. Creagh, E.M.; Sheehan, D. and Cotter, T.G. (2000). Heat shock proteins-modulators of apoptosis in tumour cells. *Leukemia*, **14**: 1161-1173.

19. De Maio, A. (1999). Heat shock proteins: facts, thoughts, and dreams. *Shock (Augusta, Ga.)*, 11(1): 1–12.

20. Donnay, I.; Feugang, J.M.; Bernard, S.; Marchandise, J.; Pampfer, S.; Moens, A. and Dessy, F. (2002). Impact of adding 5.5 mM glucose to SOF medium on the development, metabolism and quality of *in vitro* produced bovine embryos from the morula to the blastocyst stage. *Zygote*, **10**(3): 189-199.

21. Dutt, R.H. (1961). Temperature and light as factors in reproduction among farm animals. *J. Dairy Sci.*, **43**: 123-144.

22. Ealy, A.D.; Howell, J.L.; Monterroso, V.H.; Aréchiga, C.F. and Hansen, P.J. (1995). Developmental changes in sensitivity of bovine embryos to heat shock and use of antioxidants as thermoprotectants. *J. Anim. Sci.*, **73**: 1401-1407.

23. Edwards, J.L. and Hansen, P.J. (1996). Elevated temperature increases heat shock protein 70 synthesis in bovine two-cell embryos and compromises function of maturing oocyte. *Biol. Reprod.*, **55**: 340-346.

24. Edwards, J.L. and Hansen, P.J. (1997). Differential responses of bovine oocytes and preimplantation embryos to heat shock. *Mol. Reprod. Dev.*, **46**: 138-145.

25. Edwards, J.L.; Ealy, A.D.; Monterroso, V.H. and Hansen, P.J. (1997).Ontogeny of temperature-regulated heat shock protein 70 synthesis in pre-implantation bovine embryos. *MolReprod Develop.*, **48**: 25-33.

26. Edwards, J.L.; Saxton, A.N.; Lawrence, J.L.; Payton, R.R. and Dunlap, J.R. (2005). Exposure to a physiologically relevant elevated temperature hastens *in vitro* maturation of bovine oocytes. *J. Diary Sci.*, **88**: 4326-4333.

27. Eppig, J.J.; O'Brien, M. and Wigglesworth, K. (1996). Mammalian oocyte growth and development *in vitro*. *Mol. Reprod. Develop.*,**44**: 260-273.

28. Eyestone, W.H.; Jones, J.M. and First, N.L. (1991). Some factors affecting the efficacy of oviduct tissue-conditioned medium for the culture of early bovine embryos. *J. Reprod. Fertil.*, **92**(1): 59-64.

29. Ferreira, E.M.; Vireque, A.A.; Adona, P.R.; Meirelles, F.V.; Ferriani, R.A. and Navarro, P.A. (2009). Cytoplasmic maturation of bovine oocytes: structural and biochemical modifications and acquisition of developmental competence. *Theriogenology*, **71**: 836-848.

30. Finch, V.A. (1986). Body-emperature in beef cattle- Its control and relevance to production in the tropics. *J. Anim. Sci.*, **62**(2): 531-542.

31. Fissore, R.A.; Kurokawa, M.; Knott, J.; Zhang, M. and Smyth, J. (2002). Mechanism underlying oocyte activation and postovulatory aging. *Reprod.*, **124**: 745-754.

32. Fukui, Y.; McGowan, L.T.; James, R.W.; Pugh, P.A. and Tervit, H.R. (1991). Factors affecting the *in vitro* development to blastocysts of bovine oocytes matured and fertilized *in vitro*. *J. Reprod. Fertil.*, **92**(1): 125-131.

33. Fuse, T.; Yoon, K.W.; Kato, T. and Yamada, K. (1998). Heat-induced apoptosis in human glioblastoma cell line A172. *Neurosurgery*, **42**: 843–849.

34. Garcia-Ispierto, I.; Lopez-Gatius, F.; Santolaria, P.; Yaniz, J.L.; Nogareda, C.; Lopez-Bejar, M. and De Rensis, F. (2006). Relationship between heat stress during the preimplantation period and early fetal loss in dairy cattle. *Theriogenelogy*, **65**(4): 799-807.

35. Gardner, D.K.; Pool, T.B. and Lane, M. (2000). Embryo nutrition and energy metabolism and its relationship to embryo growth, differentiation, and viability. *Reprod. Med.*, **18**(2): 205-218.

36. Hansen, P.J. (2009). Effects of heat stress on mammalian reproduction. *Phil. Trans. R. Soc. B.*, **364**: 3341–3350.

37. Hansen, P.J. (2013). Cellular and molecular basis of therapies to ameliorate effects of heat stress on embryonic development in cattle. *Anim. Reprod.*, **10**(3): 322-333.

38. Hyttel, P.; Fair, T.; Callesen, H. and Greve, T. (1997). Oocyte growth, capacitation and final maturation in cattle. *Theriogenology*, **47**: 23-32.

39. Ingraham, R.H; Stanley, R.W. and Wagner, W.C. (1976). Relationship of temperature and humidity to conception rate of Holstein cows in Hawaii. *J. Dairy Sci.*, **59**: 2086-2090.

40. Ishikawa, T.; Igarashi, T.; Hata, K. and Fujita, T. (1999). *c-fos*induction by heat, arsenite, and cadmium is mediated by a heat shock element in its promoter. *Biochem. Biophys. Res. Commun.*, **254**: 566-571.

41. Jaattela, M. (1999). Heat shock proteins as cellular lifeguards. *Ann. Med.*, **31**: 261-271.

42. Johnson, H.D.; Ragsdale, A.C.; Berry, I.L. and Shanklin, M.D. (1962). Effect of various temperature-humidity combinations on milk production of Holstein cattle. *Missour. Agric. Exp. Stn. Res. Bull.*, **791**: 1-39.

43. Ju, J.C. (2005). Cellular responses of oocytes and embryos under thermal stress: hints to molecular signalling. *Anim. Reprod.*, **2**(2): 79-90.

44. Ju, J.C. and Tseng, J.K. (2004). Nuclear and cytoskeletal alterations of *in vitro* matured porcine oocytes under hyperthermia. *Mol. Reprod. Develop.*, **68**: 125-133.

45. Ju, J.C.; Parks, J.E. and Yang, X. (1999). Thermotolerance of IVM-derived bovine oocytes and embryos after short-term heat shock. *Mol. Reprod. Develop.*, **53**: 336-340.

46. Killian G.J. (2004). Evidence for the role of oviduct secretions in sperm function, fertilization and embryo development. *Anim. Reprod. Sci.*, **82-83**: 141-153.

47. Krisher, R.L. and Bavister, B.D. (1998). Responses of oocytes and embryos to the culture environment. *Theriogenology.*, **49**: 103-114.

48. Kunavongkrit, A.; Suriyasomboon, A.; Lundeheim, N. Heard, T.W. and Einarsson, S. (2005). Management and sperm production of boars under differing environmental conditions. *Theriogenology*, **63**: 657-667.

49. Kurowicka, B.; Gajewska, A. and Franczak, A. (2006). Effect of early thermal experience on pituitary-gonadal axis in female rats. *Reprod. Biol.*, **6**: 63-77.

50. Lawrence, J.L.; Payton, R.R.; Godkin, J.D.; Saxton, A.M.; Schrick, F.N. and Edwards, J.L. (2004). Retinol improves development of bovine oocytes compromised by heat stress during maturation. *J. Dairy Sci.*, **87**(8): 2449-2454.

51. Lee, D.H. (1965). Climatic stress indices for domestic animals. *Int. J. Biometorol.*, **9**(1): 29-35.

52. Lenz, R.W.; Ball, G.D.; Leibfried, M.L.; Ax, R.L. and First, N.L. (1983). *In vitro* maturation and fertilization of bovine oocytes are temperature-dependant processes. *BiolReprod.*, **29**: 173-179.

53. Levesque, J.T. and Sirard, M.A. (1996). Resumption of meiosis is initiated by the accumulation of cyclin B in bovine oocytes. *Biol. Reprod.*, **55**: 1427-1436.

54. Lindquist, S. (1986).The heat shock response.*Annu. Rev. Biochem.*, **55**: 1151-1191.

55. Mathias, S.; Pena, L.A. and Kolesnick, R.N. (1998). Signal transduction of stress via ceramide. Ceramide also plays a pivotal role in stress-induced apoptosis. *Biochem. J.*, **335**: 465-480.

56. Maya-Soriano, M.J. (2012).Heat Stress and Antioxidant Agents Effects on Gamete Development. PhD Dissertation, UniverstatAutonoma de Barcelona, Spain.

57. Merton, J. S.; de Roos,A. P.; Mullaart, E.; de Ruigh, L.; Kaal, L.; Vos, P.L. and Dieleman, S.J. (2003). Factors affecting oocyte quality and quantity in commercial application of embryo technologies in the cattle breeding industry. *Theriogenology*, **59**(2): 651-667.

58. Monty, D.E. and Racowsky, C. (1987). *In vitro* evaluation of early embryo viability and development in summer heat-stressed,superovulated dairy cows. *Theriogenology*, **28**: 451-465.

59. Moor, R.M.; Smith, M.W. and Dawson, M.C. (1980). Measurement of intercellular coupling between oocyte and cumulus cells using intracellular markers. *Exp. Cell Res.*, **126**: 15-29.

60. Mosser, D.D.; Caron, A.W.; Bourget, L.; Denis-Larose, C. and Massie, B. (1997). Role of human heat shock protein hsp70 in protection against heat-induced apoptosis. *Mol. Cell Biol.*, **17**: 5317–5327.

61. Myers, M.W.; Broussard, J.R.; Menezo, Y.; Prough, S.G.; Blackwell, J.; Godke, R.A. and Thibodeaux, J.K. (1994). Established cell lines and their conditioned media support bovine embryo development during in-vitro culture. *Human Reprod.*,**9**(10): 1927-1931.

62. Nabenishi, H.; Takagi, S.; Kamata, H.; Nishimoto, T.; Morita, T.; Ashizawa, K. and Tsuzuki Y. (2012). The role of mitochondrial transition pores on bovine oocyte competence after heat stress, as determined by effects of cyclosporin A. *Mol. Reprod. Dev.*, **79**: 31-40.

63. Okada, A.; Inomata, K. and Nagae, T. (1993).Spontaneous cortical granule release and alteration of zonapellucida properties during and after meiotic maturation of mouse oocytes. *Anat Rec.*, **237**: 518-526.

64. Parsell, D.A. and Lindquist, S. (1993). The function of heat shock proteins in stress tolerance: degradation and reactivation of damaged proteins. *Annu. Rev. Genet.*, **27**: 437-496.

65. Patriarca, E.J. and Maresca, B. (1990). Acquired thermotolerance following heat-shock protein-synthesis prevents impairment of mitochondrial ATPase activity at elevated temperature in *Saccharomyces cerevisiae*. *Exp. Cell Res.*, **190**(1): 57-64.

66. Paula-Lopes, F.F. and Hansen, P.J. (2002a). Heat-shock induced apoptosis in bovine preimplantation embryos is a developmentally-regulated phenomenon. *BiolReprod.*, **66**: 1169–1177.

67. Paula-Lopes, F.F. and Hansen, P.J. (2002b). Apoptosis is an adaptive response in bovine preimplantation embryos that facilitates survival after heat shock. *Biochem. Biophys. Res. Commun.*, **295**: 37–42.

68. Payton, R.R.; Lawrence, J.L.; Saxton, A.M.; Dunlap, J.R. and Edwards, J.L. (2003). Cortical granule types and nuclear stage of bovine oocytes after exposure to elevated temperature during maturation. *Theriogenology*, **59**: 496.

69. Payton, R.R.; Romar, R.; Coy, P.; Saxton, A.M.; Lawrence, J.L. and Edwards, J.L. (2004). Susceptibility of bovine germinal vesicle-stage oocytes from antral follicles to direct effects of heat stress *in vitro*. *Biol. Reprod.*, **71**: 1303-1308.

70. Perreault, S.D.; Barbee, R.R. and Slott, V.L. (1988). Importance of glutathione in the acquisition and maintenance of sperm nuclear decondensing activity in maturing hamster oocytes. *Develop. Biol.*, **125**: 181–186.

71. Picton, H.; Briggs, D. and Gosden, R. (1998).The molecular basis of oocyte growth and development.*Mol. Cell. Endocrinol.*, **145**: 27–37.

72. Pincus, G. and Enzmann, E.V. (1935).The comparative behavior of mammalian eggs *in vivo* and *in vitro*- I. The activation of ovarian eggs. *J. Expt. Med.*, **62**: 665-675.

73. Piper, P.W.; Millson, S.H.; Mollapour, M.; Panaretou, B.; Siligardi, G.; Pearl, L.H. and Prodromou, C. (2003). Sensitivity to Hsp90-targeting drugs can arise with mutation to the Hsp90 chaperone, cochaperones and plasma membrane ATP binding cassette transporters of yeast. *Eur. J. Biochem.*, **270**(23): 4689-4695.

74. Putney, D.J.; Mullins, S.; Thatcher, W.W.; Drost, M. and Gross, T.S. (1989). Embryonic development in superovulated dairy cattle exposed to elevated ambient temperatures between the onset of estrus and insemination. *Anim. Reprod. Sci.*, 19: 37-51.

75. Rivera, R.M.; Kelly, K.L.; Erdos, G.W. and Hansen, P.J. (2004). Reorganization of microfilaments and microtubules by thermal stress in two-cell bovine embryos. *Biol. Reprod.*, **70**: 1852-1862.

76. Roth, Z. and Hansen, P.J. (2004). Involvement of apoptosis in disruption of developmental competence of bovine oocytes by heat shock during maturation. *Biol. Reprod.*, **71**: 1898–1906.

77. Roth, Z. and Hansen, P.J. (2005). Disruption of nuclear maturation and rearrangement of cytoskeletal elements in bovine oocytes exposed to heat shock during maturation. *Reprod.*, **129**: 235-244.

78. Roth, Z.; Arav, A.; Bor, A.; Zeron, Y. Braw-Tal, R. and Wofenson, D. (2001). Improvement of quality of oocytes collected in the autumn by enhanced removal of impaired follicles from previously heat-stressed cows. *Reprod.*,**122**: 737-744.

79. Rozenboim, I.; Tako, E.; Gal-Garber, O.; Proudman, J.A. and Uni, Z. (2007). The effect of heat stress on ovarian function of laying hens. *Poultry Sci.*, **86**: 1760-1765.

80. Schrock, G.E.; Saxton, A.M.; Shrick, F.N. and Edwards, J.L. (2007). Early *in vitro* fertilization improves development of bovine ova heat stressed during *in vitro* maturation. *J. Dairy Sci.*, **90**: 4297-4303.

81. Shimizu, T.; Ohshima, I.; Ozawa, M.; Takahashi, S.; Tajima, A.; Shiota, M.; Miyazaki, H. and Kanai, Y. (2005). Heat stress diminishes gonadotropin receptor expression and enhances susceptibility to apoptosis to rat granulosa cells. *Reprod.*, **129**: 463-472.

82. Sirard, M.A. (2001). Resumption of meiosis: mechanism involved in meiotic progression and its relation with developmental competence. *Theriogenology*, **55**: 1241-1254.

83. Sonna, L.A.; Fujita, J.; Gaffan, S.L. and Lilly, C.M. (2002). Molecular Biology of Thermoregulation Invited Review: Effects of heat and cold stress on mammalian gene expression. *J. App. Physio.*, **92**: 1725-42.

84. Soto, P. and Smith, L.C. (2009). BH4 peptide derived from Bcl-xL and Bax-inhibitor peptide suppresses apoptotic mitochondrial changes in heat stressed bovine oocytes. *Mol. Reprod. Develop.*, **76**: 637-646.

85. Stojkovic, M.; Machado, S.A.; Stojkovic, P.; Zakhartchenko, V.; Hutzler, P.; Goncalves, P.B. and Wolf, E. (2001). Mitochondrial distribution and adenosine triphosphate content of bovine oocytes before and after *in vitro* maturation: correlation with morphological criteria and developmental capacity after *in vitro* fertilization and culture. *Biol. Reprod.*, **64**: 904-909.

86. Streffer, C. (1984). Mechanism of heat injury. In: *Hyperthermic Oncology*. Overgaard J. (Editor). London: Taylor and Francis, pp. 213-222.

87. Sugiyama, G.; McGowan, M.; Phillips, N.; Kafi, M. and Young, M. (2007). Effects of increased ambient temperature during IVM and/ or IVF on the *in vitro* development of bovine zygotes. *Reprod. Domest. Anim.*, **42**: 271-274.

88. Takahashi, T.; Takahashi, E.; Igarashi, H.; Tezuka, N. and Kurachi, H. (2003). Impact of oxidative stress in aged mouse oocytes on calcium oscillations at fertilization. *Mol. Reprod. Develop.*, **66**: 143-152.

89. Tanghe, S.; Van Soom, A.; Nauwynck, H.; Coryn, M. and de Kruif, A. (2002). Minireview: functions of the cumulus oophorus during oocyte maturation, ovulation, and fertilization. *Mol. Reprod. Develop.*, **61**: 414-424.

90. Tarin, J.J.; Vendrell, F.J.; Ten, J.; Blanes, R. van Blerkom, J. and Cano, A. (1996). The oxidizing agent tertiary butyl hydroperoxide induces disturbances in spindle organization, c-meiosis and aneuploidy in mouse oocytes. *Mol. Human Reprod.*, **2**(12): 895-901.

91. Tatemoto, H.; Sakuri, N. and Muto, N. (2000). Protection of porcine oocytes against apoptotic cell death caused by oxidative stress during *in vitro* maturation: role of cumulus cells. *Biol. Reprod.*, **63**: 805-810.

92. Thibault, C. (1966). La culture *In vitro* de I'oeuf de vache. *Ann. Biol. Anim. Biochim. Biophys.*, **7**: 5-23.

93. Thom, E.C. (1959). The discomfort index. *Weatherwise*, **12**(1): 57-60.

94. Thompson, J.G. (2000). *In vitro* culture and embryo metabolism of cattle and sheep embryos - a decade of achievement. *Anim. Reprod. Sci.*, **60-61**: 263-275.

95. Toivola, D.M.; Strnad, P.; Habtezion, A. and Omary, M.B. (2010). Intermediate filaments take the heat as stress proteins. *Trends Cell Biol.*, **20**(2): 79-91.

96. Torres-Junior, J.R.D.; Pires, M.D.A.; De Sa, W.F.; Feffeira, A.D.; Viana, J.H.M.; Camargo, L.S.A.; Ramos, A.A.; Folhadella, I.M.; Polisseni, J.; de Freitas, C.; Clemente, C.A.A.; De Sa, M.F.; Paula-Lopez, F.F. and Baruselli, P.D. (2008). Effect of maternal heat stress on follicular growth and oocyte competence in *Bosindicus* cattle. *Theriogenology*, **69**(2): 155-166.

97. Tseng, J.K. (2004). Nuclear and cytoskeletal alterations of *in vitro* matured porcine oocytes under hyperthermia. *Mol. Reprod. Develop.*, **68**: 125-133.

98. Tseng, J.K.; Tang, P.C. and Ju, J.C. (2006). *In vitro* thermal stress induces apoptosis and reduces development of porcine parthenotes. *Theriogenology*, **66**(5): 1073-1082.

99. Vigh, L.; Nakamoto, H.; Landry, J.; Gomez-Munoz, A.; Harwood, J.L. and Hovarth, I. (2007). Membrane regulation of the stress response from prokaryotic models to mammalian cells. *Ann. NY Acad. Sci.*, **1113**: 40-51.

100. Wang, J.Z.; Sui, H.S.; Miao, D.Q.; Liu, N.; Zhou, P. Ge, L. and Tan, J.H. (2008). Effects of stress during *in vitro* maturation of cytoplasmic versus nuclear components of mouse oocytes. *Reprod.*, **137**: 1-10.

101. Warnes, G.M.; Moor, R.M. and Johnson, M.H. (1977). Changes in protein synthesis during maturation of sheep oocytes *in vivo* and *in vitro*. *J. Reprod.Fertil.*, **49**: 331-335.

102. Welch, W. and Suhan, J. (1985). Morphological study of the mammalian stress response characterization of changes in cytoplasmic organelles, cytoskeleton, and nucleoli, and appearance of intranuclear actin filaments in rat fibroblast after heat shock treatment. *J Cell Biol.*, **101**: 1198-1211.

103. Wolfenson, D.; Lew, B.J.; Thatcher, W.W.; Graber, Y. and Meidan, R. (1997). Seasonal and acute heat stress effects on steroid production by dominant follicles in cows. *Anim. Reprod. Sci.*, **47**: 9-19.

104. Wrzal, P. (2006). Molecular Mechanisms of Apoptosis Activation by Heat Shock in Multidrug-Resistant Chinese Hamster Cells Overexpressing P-Glycoprotein. Ph.D. Thesis. Université Du Québec À Montréal.

105. Yuan, Y,Q,; Van Soom, A.; Coopman, F.J.; Mintiens, K.; Boerjan, M.L.; Van Zeveren, A.; De Kruif, A. and Peelman, L.J. (2003). Influence of oxygen tension on apoptosis and hatching in bovine embryos cultured *in vitro*. *Theriogenology*, **59**: 1585-1596.

106. Yuan, Y.; Hao, Z.D.; Liu, J.; Wu, Y.; Yang, L.; Liu, G.S.; Tian, J.H.; Zhu, S.E. and Zeng, S.M. (2008). Heat shock at the germinal vesicle breakdown stage induces apoptosis in surrounding cumulus cells and reduces maturation rates of porcine oocytes *in vitro*. Theriogenology, **70**(2): 168-178.

107. Zeron, Y.; Ocheretny, A.; Kedar, O.; Borochov, A.; Sklan, D. and Arav, A. (2001). Seasonal changes in bovine fertility: relation to oocyte developmental competence, membrane properties and follicle fatty acid composition. *Reprod.*, **121**: 447-454.

108. Zhang, L.; Jiang, S.; Wozniak, P.J.; Yang, X. and Godke, R.A. (1995). Cumulus cell function during bovine oocyte maturation, fertilization and embryo development *in vitro*. *Mol. Reprod. Develop.*, **40**(3): 338-344.

109. Zimbelman, R.B.; Rhoads, R.P.; Rhoads, M.L.; Duff, G.C.; Baunmgard, L.H. and Collier, R.J. (2009). A re-evaluation of the impact of Temperature Humidity Index (THI) and Black Globe Humidity Index (BGHI) on milk production in high producing dairy cows. Proceedings of the American Registry of Professional Animal Scientists, Southwest Nutrition and Management Conference, pp. 26-27.

❑❑❑

Chapter 3

Genome Editing : A Challenging way for Sustainable Livestock Species Development

A. K. DAS, RAJIB DEB AND GYANENDRA SINGH SENGAR

ICAR-Central Institute for Research on Cattle, Meerut-250 001, UP, India

Introduction

Genome editing is the process of editing an organisms DNA by altering, removing or adding nucleotides to the genome (Bogdanove & Voytas, 2011; van der Oost, *et al.*, 2013). This process is accomplished through the use of engineered nucleases that can make a double stranded "cut" or a single stranded "nick" in an organism's DNA. These sites are altered and then repaired by homologous recombination or non-homologous end joining. This type of genetic engineering is useful for a number of applications, including targeted gene mutations, chromosomal rearrangement, and the creation of transgenic animals.

The agricultural application of genetic engineering has advanced in the field of crop breeding. In 1994, the US Food and Drug Administration (FDA) approved a genetically modified (GM) tomato variety, the world's first GM crop for food consumption (Bruening and Lyons, 2000). In this GM tomato (the FlavrSavr), ripening was delayed by the insertion of an antisense gene that interferes with polygalacturonase production. Although the regulatory approval of GM crops largely demands strict assessments of the environmental risks and food safety, the commercial cultivation of GM crops with an exogenous gene (termed transgene) has spread to at least 28 countries, including the USA, Brazil, Argentina, India, Canada, China, and some European countries (Ishii and Araki, 2016). Conversely, there have been few regulatory approvals regarding GM livestock, with the exception of GM goats for "pharming" in which biopharmaceuticals are manufactured using transgenesis (FDA, 2009). Currently, older genetic engineering practices, such as transgenesis, are giving way to genome editing. Genome editing tools, such as zincfinger nucleases (ZFNs; Klug, 2010), transcription activator-like effector nucleases (TALENs; Joung and Sander, 2013), and the clustered regularly interspaced short palindromic repeat (CRISPR)/Cas 9 (Barrangou and Doudna, 2016), can break DNA double strands at target sites and then achieve various types of genetic modification via non-homologous end-joining (NHEJ) or homology-directed repair (HDR), thus potentially adding new value to agriculture (Fig. 1). Recent reviews suggest that NHEJ is preferred in crop genome editing because the resultant plants are considered to contain no transgenes, which is one of the major concerns over GM crops from regulatory and social aspects (Hartung and Schiemann, 2014; Voytas and Gao, 2014; Araki and Ishii, 2015). Genome editing has also been applied in livestock breeding (Carlson *et al.*, 2012; Hai *et al.*, 2014; Crispo *et al.*, 2015; Cui *et al.*, 2015; Proudfoot *et al.*, 2015; Wang *et al.*, 2015a; Wang *et al.*, 2015b; Wang *et al.*, 2015c; Carlson *et al.*, 2016; Fischer *et al.*, 2016; Oishi *et al.*, 2016; Petersen *et al.*, 2016; Tanihara *et al.*, 2016; Wang *et al.*, 2016; Whitworth *et al.*, 2016). Animals modified via NHEJ are unlikely to impose substantial risks on the environment because they can be managed within a farm, unlike GM crops, which are intentionally released into the environment (field cultivation). Thus, one can presume that the products derived from genome-edited livestock will soon be accepted in society if the food safety can be confirmed. However, it would be inappropriate to presume that such a favourable course of events is the only possibility. In November 2015, the FDA approved a GM salmon for food consumption (FDA, 2015). Nonetheless, citizen groups and environmentalists still loudly oppose the FDA's decision about its safety. In addition, they questioned the environmental risk that it posed to wild salmon populations; despite that the sterile GM fish is only raised in landlocked tanks (Pollack, 2015). Such public movements may have prolonged the FDA review of the GM salmon. It took nearly a quarter of a century and cost more than \$77 million (Van Eenennaam and Muir, 2011). Psychological investigations have suggested that GM animals are viewed as less acceptable than GM plants and that people's sense of ethics has a more significant effect on the acceptance than other factors such as the perceived risks, the recognized benefits, or the trust in regulators and researchers (Zechendorf, 1994; Siegrist, 2000). Likewise, complex situations are likely to emerge in the case of livestock genome editing because animals modified via NHEJ are also genetically modified.

Historical Background of Genome Editing

Genome editing has been a heavily studied field for a number of years with an ultimate goal of specificity to limit off target effects. The first engineered nuclease technology, Zinc Finger, was presented in a 1991 publication by Pavletich and Pabo in the journal Science. Zinc Finger was the predominant genome targeting technology for over ten years, but over time drawbacks to the system emerged. Certain nucleotide triplets could not be targeted, and interactions within a zinc finger array could reduce specificity.

In 2009 when the genome targeting abilities of TAL effectors was published, they were quickly harnessed for genome editing and transcription activator-like effector nuclease, or TALEN, emerged. TALEN allowed for a larger window of potential target sites and a simple method of building TAL effector arrays was introduced in 2011. As a result of these advancements and its overall potential, TALEN was named "Method of the Year 2011" by the journal nature methods.

In 2012, clustered regularly interspaced short palindromic repeats, or CRISPR, was demonstrated as a new genome editing tool. CRISPR was discovered somewhat fortuitously by researchers studying bacterial defense mechanisms, specifically how bacteria deal with foreign plasmids and phages. Bacteria have the ability to open and alter the genomes of invading viruses with a nuclease called Cas9, inactivating them in the process. CRISPR formulates a complex containing the Cas9 nuclease and small guide RNAs (sgRNA) and can be redirected by using different sgRNAs. This property eliminates the need to construct a completely customized endonuclease for each target, something that is still required by TALEN and Zinc Finger. As a result of this the entry barrier to genome editing has been lowered significantly, allowing for more users and more innovation.

Mechanisms of Genome Editing

Two genome editing technologies have emerged recently that exploit bacterial systems for plant pathogenesis or adaptive immunity: TALEN (Transcription Activator-Like Effector Nucleases) and CRISPR (Clustered, Regularly Interspaced, Short Palindromic Repeats), respectively. Both TALEN and CRISPR use endonucleases that initiate double-strand breaks (DSBs) at virtually any genomic target sequence, and are used for many applications, including gene knockout, transgene knock-in, gene tagging, and correction of genetic defects.

Genome editing starts with efficient DSB generation in the target DNA (Fig. 1). DSBs are repaired either by homologous recombination (HR), or, in the absence of a homologous repair template, via non-homologous end joining (NHEJ). NHEJ causes small insertions or deletions as the broken ends are pieced back together. This proclivity for indel generation is exploited as a convenient method for knocking genes out. Both TALEN, which is comprised of a pair of DNA binding proteins fused to the FokI nuclease, and CRISPR, which is a complex between the Cas9 nuclease and a target-specific single guide RNA (sgRNA), can edit DNA through either HR or NHEJ.

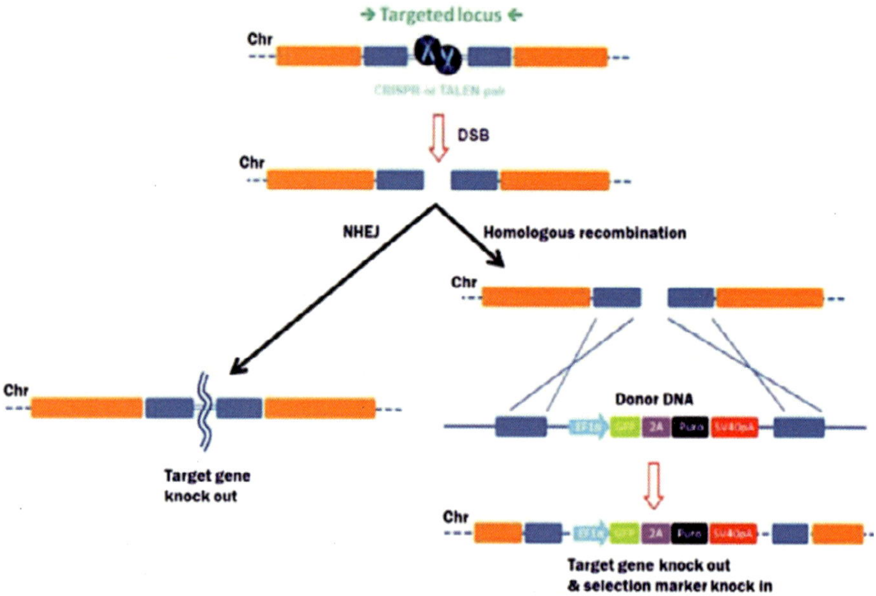

Fig. 1. Pathways for repair of DSBs induced by genome editing tools. Left: Non-homologous end joining. Right : Homologous recombination in the presence of a donor template. http://www.genecopoeia.com/product/genome-editing/.

Genome Edition by Nucleases

In the last decade, new methodologies of genome manipulation have emerged. A series of custom target nucleases with the ability to specifically target the genomic region of interest and cleave the phosphodiester bonds have been developed (Urnov *et al.*, 2005, Miller *et al.*, 2007, Christian *et al.*, 2010, Miller *et al.*, 2010, Kim and Kim 2014). The broad concept underlying the new genome editing tools is that by stimulating DNA double-strand breaks (DSBs) at a target region, the endogenous repair machinery of the cell could be hijacked to introduce targeted mutations. In the absence of a homologous repair template, InDels (insertions/deletions) may occur via error-prone non-homologous end joining (NHEJ). These may alter the open reading frame (ORF) of the target gene leading to a premature stop codon or translation of a scrambled amino acid sequence. Notably, the InDels induced by NHEJ are random, therefore the outcome cannot be predicted (Bibikova *et al.*, 2002, Sander and Joung 2014). The generation of In Dels within a mutated genomic region may also restore gene function through the correction of disease causing mutations (Long, McAnally *et al.*, 2014). Therefore, the engineered nucleases to be described in the next sessions, Zinc-finger nucleases (ZFNs), Transcription Activator-Like Effector Nucleases (TALENs) and CRISPR-Cas systems, allowed the generation of transgenic organisms in a more efficient way and have introduced a new era in gene function analysis (Fig. 2).

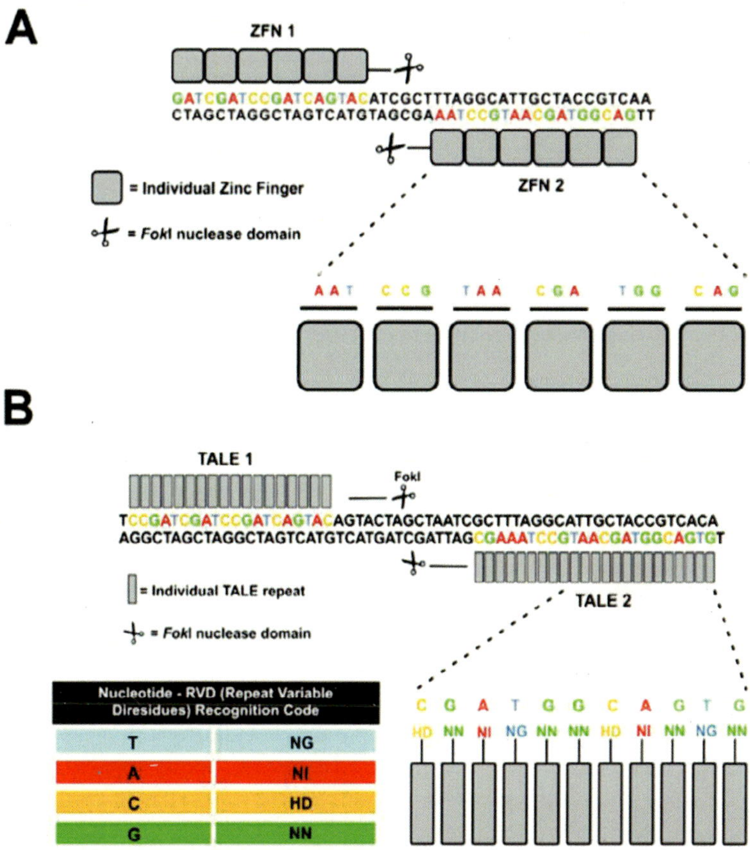

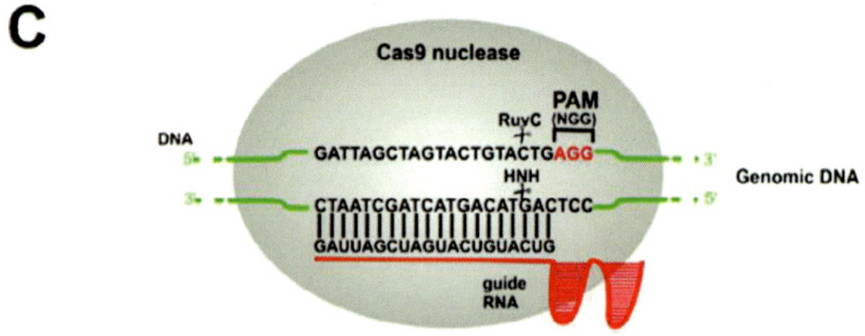

Fig. 2. Molecular mechanisms of DNA recognition: ZFNs, TALENs and CRISPR/Cas9

(A) Illustration of a ZFN pair bound to DNA sequence on opposite strands. In this case, each individual zinc finger domain (gray square) binds to a nucleotide triplet. (B) Illustration of a TALEN pair bound to DNA sequence on opposite strands. Note that each individual TALEN module (gray rectangle) is bound to a specific nucleotide, through interactions of two amino acid residues (RVD - repeat variable diresidues) and the nucleotide (inset in TALEN 2). The RVD-nucleotide recognition code is shown on the left. The FokI DNA cleavage domains of each ZFN (A) or TALEN (B) are juxtaposed and present a spacer region in between them. (C) The CRISPR/Cas9 recognition system consists of a guide RNA (gRNA, red) transcript and the Cas9 nuclease. The gRNA requires an adjourning NGG sequence (PAM) for Cas9 recognition and directs DNA cleavage through base pair complementarity. Ruv C and HNH nuclease domains of Cas9 create DSBs at the genomic target site (green). (Anais da Academia Brasileira de Ciências (2015) 87 (2 Suppl.) : 1323-1348).

Protein-guided Engineered Nucleases

The use of ZFNs (Zinc-Finger Nucleases) and TALENs (Transcription Activator-Like Effector Nucleases) facilitated the generation of transgenic animals. In comparison to the endogenous DNA break events, the activity of the engineered nucleases may increase the frequency of DSBs in a specific region in about 10,000-100,000 (Moehle *et al.*, 2007). In addition to ZFNs and TALENs, other valuable tools for genome editing have been developed (e.g. meganucleases and transposons). One of the biggest limitations imposed by restriction endonucleases was the small size of the DNA site to be recognized, what hampered their use when working with larger DNA sequences due to cleavage activity in multiple sites. Also, most restriction enzymes present DNA binding and cleavage activity within the same domain, limiting their targeting capability (Lanio *et al.,* 2000). However, a few of them have separate binding and cleavage domains, such as *Fok*I. In order to increase the possible binding sites for restriction enzymes, Dr. Srinivasan Chandrasegaran and colleagues envisioned an approach of linking DNA binding region of homeodomain transcription factors to the cleavage domain of *Fok*I. The resultant artificial nuclease contained a DNA binding homeodomain fused to *Fok*I nuclease, being able to cleave DNA sequences nearby homeodomain-binding sites (Kim and Chandrasegaran 1994). Later on, this same group assembled the first ZFNs (Kim *et al.,* 1996), paving the way to genome tailoring at custom sites.

ZFNs are chimeric proteins composed of a modular array of Cys2-His2 DNA-binding zinc fingers fused to a *Fok*I nuclease domain (Kim *et al.,* 1996, Bibikova *et al.,* 2001, Urnov *et al.,* 2010). These modular arrays are usually composed of 3-6 zinc fingers that recognize three nucleotides each, providing DNA binding specificity to the nuclease (Greisman and Pabo 1997, Wolfe *et al.,* 2000, Maeder *et al.,* 2008, Ramirez, Foley *et al.,* 2008). A pair of ZFNs must be designed to target a given genomic region, since the *Fok*I nuclease domain requires dimerization to work (Bitinaite *et al.,* 1998). Each zinc finger array binds to close DNA regions, on opposite strands, so that a DSB is induced in a specific genomic site.

Similar to ZFNs, TALENs were developed by fusing the *Fok*I endonuclease domain with an array of TALE repeats. TALEN assembly is much less problematic in comparison to ZFN, although some difficulties are present. Different from ZFNs, modular assembly of TALE repeats results in the predicted DNA binding pattern. On the other hand, cloning steps to generate the desired TALEs can be challenging due to the high DNA sequence homology between the different repeats. However, advances in cloning systems are helping to overcome these difficulties (Engler *et al.,* 2008). As an example, libraries of TALENs targeting most of human coding-genes and microRNAs were recently developed (Kim *et al.,* 2013).

RNA-guided Nucleases: CRISPR/Cas9

As mentioned, a challenging aspect of the ZFN and TALE protein-guided approaches is the requirement to design new modular DNA-binding proteins for each gene target. It became clear that engineering nucleases guided by alternative modes of DNA recognition would simplify genome editing. At this point, the RNA-guided endonuclease technology CRISPR/Cas9 is established as the less time-consuming method of reduced cost that allows targeting of multiple DNA sites. These features brought the possibility of transgenesis at a system level one step closer (Cong *et al.*, 2013, Mali *et al.*, 2013).

The development of the Cas9 endonuclease for genome editing became possible due to more than a decade of research on the biological function of the repetitive elements now known as CRISPR (clustered regularly interspaced short palindromic repeats). A study on the chromosomal DNA segment that contains iap gene in *E. coli*, an enzyme responsible for isozyme conversion of alkaline phosphatase, reported an unusual series of repeat sequences (direct repeats) interspaced by variable sequences (spacers) (Ishino *et al.*, 1987). Sequencing of other microbial genomes revealed that these interspaced repeat sequences were present across many species (~40% of sequenced bacteria and ~90% of archaea) and these were classified as a unique family of clustered repeat elements (Mojica *et al.*, 2000).

Despite the detailed mapping and annotation of CRISPR loci, their role remained elusive. Some suggested that the spacers descend from foreign genetic elements, such as bacteriophages (Bolotin *et al.*, 2005, Mojica *et al.*, 2005, Pourcel *et al.*, 2005). In 2007, Horvath and colleagues demonstrated that CRISPR spacers dictated target specificity through base-pair complementarities between nucleic acids, while Cas enzymes were required for the acquisition of new spacer sequences and defense from phage infection (Barrangou *et al.*, 2007).

As expected, one major concern when using CRISPR/Cas9 system is the occurrence of high off-target mutagenesis, since gRNA-DNA target binding tolerate up to three mismatches (Cradick *et al.*, 2013, Pattanayak *et al.*, 2013). In order to improve specificity without compromising on-target cleavage efficiency, Cas9 was converted to a nicking enzyme. Individual nicks in the genome are repaired with high fidelity, and simultaneous nicking by using a pair of gRNAs is necessary to effectively introduce targeted DSBs. In this case, the increase in the number of specifically recognized bases in the target site minimized the off-target activity (Ren *et al.*, 2013). Specificity can be further tuned by titration of CRISPR/Cas9 components and reduction of the regions responsible for target complementarity (spacer region) (Hsu *et al.*, 2013, Fu *et al.*, 2014). Truncated gRNAs composed by shorter spacer regions (<20 nucleotides) display less non-specific cleavage activity mutagenesis without compromising on-target activity

(Fu *et al.,* 2014). Even without undesired DSBs, a screening process is required, since the InDels induced by NHEJ repair pathway are still random.

The CRISPR/Cas9 technology was rapidly applied for gene modification in a variety of experimental model systems (*Caenorhabditis elegans* (Dickinson *et al.,* 2013), *Drosophila melanogaster* (Gratz *et al.,* 2013), *Arabidopsis thaliana* (Jiang *et al.,* 2013), *Rattusnorvegicus* (Ma *et al.,* 2013), *Danio rerio* (Hwang *et al.,* 2013), and *Macacafascicularis* (Niu *et al.,* 2014) due to advantages over other genome editing methods (Table I) (Meckler *et al.,* 2013). Cas9 and gRNA can be microinjected into embryos through the use of plasmid expression vectors or *in vitro* transcribed RNA (Hsu *et al.,* 2013, Fei *et al.,* 2014, Fujihara and Ikawa 2014, Niu *et al.,* 2014). However, generation of knockin lines expressing Cas9 nuclease, as done for mice and Drosophila, provides a straightforward method to optimize efficiency of mutagenesis and recovery of injected animals (Ren *et al.,* 2013, Platt *et al.,* 2014).

Multiplexed gene editing at unprecedented scale through a battery of short gRNAs rather than a library of large proteins is a major advantage of this approach (Cong *et al.,* 2013, Jao *et al.,* 2013, Mali *et al.,* 2013, Wang *et al.,* 2013, Ma *et al.,* 2014, Ma *et al.,* 2014, Xing *et al.,* 2014). For example, simultaneous disruption of functionally redundant genes from the same gene family (Tet1, 2, 3, Sry, Uty - 8 alleles) was accomplished in mouse ES cells. These results showed that out of 96 clones screened, 10% carried mutations in all eight alleles of the five genes (Wang *et al.,* 2013). Thus, CRISPR/ Cas9 has the potential to circumvent the need of sequential recombination and intercrossing of lines to generate animal models carrying mutations in multiple genes.

Although both ZFNs and TALENs brought advances for transgenic mice generation, drawbacks presented by whole-embryo knockin or knockout mice are still possible. As explained, some cases of embryonic lethality or organ malformation due to non-autonomous effects can be prevented by cell type/tissue-specific gene inactivation. Therefore, applications that combine engineered nucleases with other transgenesis tools, such as the Cre-*LoxP*system, can be used to reach tissue- and spatial-specificity in gene inactivation (Bedell *et al.,* 2012, Brown *et al.,* 2013) (Fig. 4).

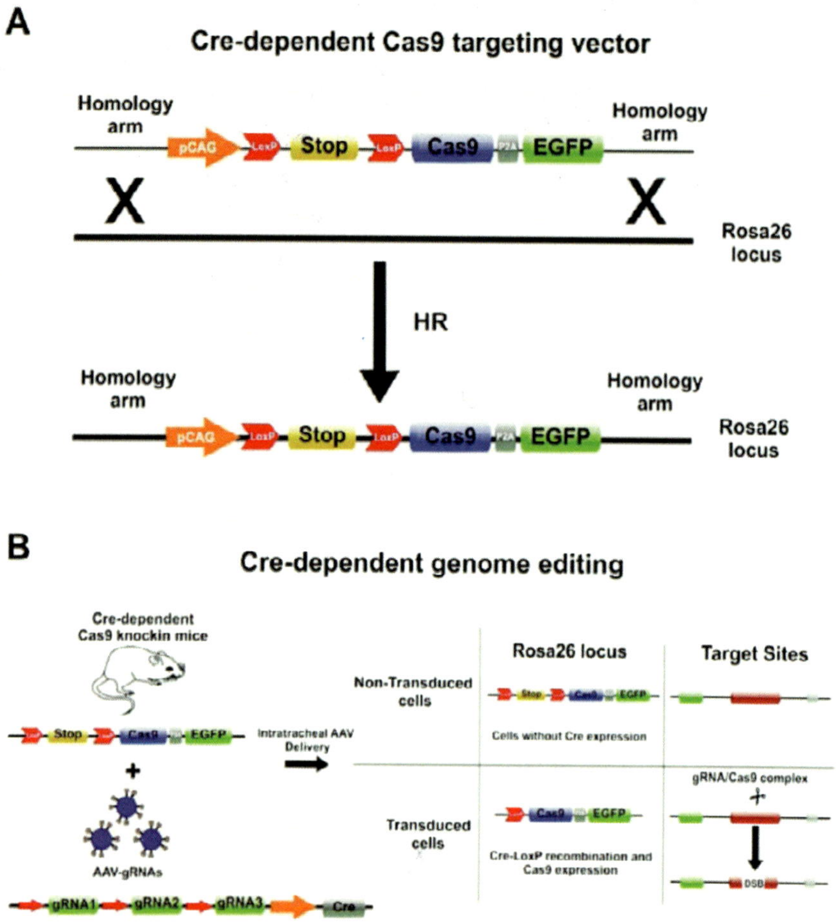

Fig. 3. Generation and applications of the Cre-Dependent Cas9 mouse knockin (A) Illustration of the Cre-dependent Cas9 Rosa26 targeting vector. Exogenous template contained ubiquitous CAG promoter (pCAG), *LoxP*-Stop-*LoxP*cassette (LSL), Cas9 nuclease gene, self-cleaving P2A peptide and the reporter gene (EGFP) flanked by two homology arms. The transgene expression cassette was introduced through homologous recombination into the Rosa26 locus. (B) Spatial and temporal control of multiplex CRISPR/Cas9-mediated genome editing. A single AAV vector integrating guide RNAs (gRNA) for three different genes as well as a Cre recombinase expression cassette was delivered into Cre-dependent Cas9 mice. In this experiment, Cre recombinase activity on transduced cells lead to excision of LSL and Cas9 expression. Cas9 nuclease activity directed by gRNAS introduce DSB at the target sites of interest. In constrast, genomic DNA of non-transduced cells remain intact, since Cas9 expression and activity relies on Cre recombinase and gRNAs, respectively. (Anais da Academia Brasileira de Ciências (2015) 87(2 Suppl.): 1323-1348)

Table 1. Comparison between different nucleases

	ZFN	TALEN	CRISPR/Cas9
Recognition mode	Protein-DNA	Protein-DNA	RNA- DNA
Recognition site	9-18 bp x 2	10-20 bp x 2	20bp
Nuclese type	Fokl	Fokl	Cas9
Size	~1 kb x 2	~3 kb x 2	~4.2 kb (Cas9) + 0.1 kb (gRNA)
Permissive mismatches	Not known	1*	3
Multiplex targeting	Very Limited	Limited	Possible (e.g. 8 alleles)
Sensitivity to DNA methylartion	Sensitive	Sensitive**	Non - Sensitive

* reported to greatly reduce cleavage activity of the TALEN (Meckler *et al.*, 2013). ** can be overcomed since TALEs recognize methylated citosines as thymines in the major groove. (*Source:* Anais da Academia Brasileira de Ciências (2015) 87(2 Suppl.): 1323-1348)

Genome Editing in Livestock

Zinc-finger nucleases and TALENs are artificial DNA cutting enzymes (nucleases) with a DNA–protein binding domain that directs the nucleases to a target sequence in the genome. CRISPR/Cas9 adopts a separate type of DNA-RNA binding system that can be readily prepared in most laboratories. Thus, the use of CRISPR/Cas9 has been particularly spreading worldwide.

The microinjection of the site-directed nucleases (in the form of plasmids, mRNAs, or proteins) into one-cell-stage animal embryos (zygotes) can effectively generate genome-edited offspring (Ishii, 2015). This approach is much simpler than GM animal production involving the transfer of embryonic stem (ES) cells into animal embryos. In addition, the one-step-generation approach is applicable even in animal species for which no ES cell line is available. This methodology has been employed for NHEJ, primarily using the cytoplasmic injection of CRISPR/Cas9 mRNA and single-guide (sg) RNA into bovine, swine, ovine, and caprine zygotes. The efficiency of genetic modification in neonates is largely high, as illustrated in the bovine [19% (Proudfoot *et al.*, 2015)], swine [50%: biallelic modification (Petersen *et al.*, 2016)], ovine [23%: homozygous KO (Crispo *et al.*, 2015)], and caprine [13%: double KO (Wang *et al.*, 2015a)] cases. Other approaches adopted

NHEJ in primordial germ cells to generate knockout fowls (Oishi *et al.*, 2016), NHEJ in somatic cells to generate double-knockout pigs via somatic cell nuclear transfer (SCNT; Fischer *et al.*, 2016), and HDR in somatic cells to develop cattle and goats in which a variant was copied or a transgene was introduced via SCNT (Wang *et al.*, 2015a; Carlson *et al.*, 2016). Overall, CRISPR/Cas9 is predominantly used in livestock genome editing. Moreover, one-step-generation via NHEJ is frequently used for gene disruption. Meanwhile, SCNT following HDR in somatic cells is applied for efficiently attaining transgenesis or copying a variant in the animal genome. Such reports have rendered precision livestock breeding technically feasible in the era of genome editing.

Genome Editing to Improve Animal Welfare

There has been an ongoing debate surrounding the dehorning of cattle. Although dehorning frequently uses invasive and laborious procedures such as disbudding and heat cauterization, it is performed worldwide to avoid causing injuries to other cattle and farm workers (Carroll *et al.*, 2016). Thus, in addition to farmers, the public are concerned about the welfare of cattle that undergo painful dehorning. A recent study described the production of a hornless strain of dairy (Holstein) cattle by copying the POLLED of beef cattle (Angus) via HDR and somatic cloning (Carlson *et al.*, 2016). The frequency of POLLED in Holstein cattle is much lower due to the small number of sires that produce commercially available POLLED semen. Therefore, this breeding could reduce the frequency of dehorning in the dairy industry,potentially enhancing the welfare of cattle.However, people are likely to contemplate the implications of the visiblechange in the cattle. Thus, some consider this visible change to represent aloss of the "essence of a creature" through genome editing. One might assert that hornless cattle are generated to prevent injury to both farmers and othercattle. However, some would still view the use of genome editing in thisregard as the initiation of "increasingly imbalanced distribution of powerbetween humans and animals" (Schicktanz, 2006). In addition, the need forthis animal genome editing would be questioned. There are alternatives:enriching the rearing environment to prevent accidents, the use of horn covers (Zen-Noh Livestock Co., 2016), and performing the dehorning of cattleunder anesthesia. It appears that the moral imperative for animals is scant in this breeding program. As a result, it is unlikely that people would accept that the use of genome editing in this setting enhances animal welfare.

Taken together, the aforementioned arguments suggest that genome editing to prevent viral infections (for the purpose of animal health) may best satisfy the animal welfare concerns and would be most acceptable under people's sense of ethics. Thus, this type of breeding may be considered for a priority program for a research group or a research institute.

Genome editing differs from older genetic engineering techniques that require the intracellular use of artificial nucleases that a researcher has designed. Some off-target mutations could be deleterious mutations that negatively affect animal health; this may lead to concerns over animal welfare. For example, missed off-target mutations could affect animal health if such unintended genetic changes lead to tumor formation due to mechanisms such as the disruption of a tumor suppressor gene. As the history of cloned animals suggests, the investigation of off-target mutations seems vital to the use of genome editing in livestock breeding from the viewpoint of animal welfare. Notably, the negative attitude of people toward GMOs is, in part, based on a lack of trust in researchers and regulators (Ishii and Araki, 2016). Thus, the further consideration of animal welfare by reducing the risk of off-target mutations might enhance people's trust and eventually foster the social acceptance of products from genome-edited livestock.

Nonetheless, there is currently no consensus regarding the means of assessing off-target mutations in genome-edited organisms (Joung, 2015). At present, it would be appropriate to investigate off-target mutations in animal embryos or somatic cells as deeply as possible, as a report on bovine genome editing demonstrated (Carlson *et al.*, 2016).

Table 2. Genome edited Livestock Species Ishii (2017)

Subject	Target Gede	Efficiency in zygotes*	Efficiency in Live Born	Off-target Mutation	Gene Editing	Delivery	Remarks	Reference
NHEJ(non-homologous end-joining)								
Bovine zygotes	MSTN	-	19%**	N.D.	TALEN	mRNA	Cytoplesmic injection	Proudfoot et al.,2015
Bovine zygotes	LDLR	3.8%	-	N.D.	TALEN	mRNA	Cytoplesmic injection	Carlson et al.,2012
Porcine zygotes	MSTN	-	20% (biallelic)	No	Cas9	Cas9 prot-ein. sgRNA	Mosaicism elecotropor-ation	Tanihara et al.,2016
Porcine zygotes	GGTAI	-	50% (biallelic)	No	Cas9	Plasmid	Mosaicism cytoplesmic injection	Petersen et al.,2016
Porcine zygotes	CD163	-	9%**	N.D.	Cas9	mRNA/ sgRNA	Cytoplesmic injection	Whirwo-rth et al., 2016
Porcine zygotes	MITF	-	5% (biallelic)**	No	Cas9	mRNA/ sgRNA	Cytoplesmic injection	Wang et al.,2015b
Porcine zygotes	Npcll	-	11%**	No	Cas9	mRNA/ sgRNA	Mosaicism cytoplesmic injection	Wang et al.,2015c
Porcine zygotes	vWF	-	15%**	No	Cas9	mRNA/ sgRNA	Cytoplesmic injection	Hai et al., 2014

Porcine zygotes	RELA	0.5%	-	N.D.	TALEN	mRNA	Cytoplesmic injection	Carison et al.,2012
Ovine zygotes	MSTN,ASIP ,BCO2	-	6% (triple KO)	No	Cas9 sgRNA	mRNA/ injection	Cytoplesmic al.,2016	Wang et
Ovine zygotes	MSTN	4.6%	23% (homo-zygous KO)	Yes (20% in mutants)	Cas9	mRNA/ sgRNA	Mosaicism cytoplesmic injection	Crispo et al., 2015
Ovine zygotes	MSTN	-	4%**	N.D.	TALEN	mRNA	Cytoplesmic injection	Proudfoot et al., 2015
Caprine zygotes	MSTN ,FGFS	-	13% (double KO)	Yes (23% in mutants)	Cas9	mRNA/ sgRNA	Cytoplesmic injection	Wang et al., 2015a
Chicken PGCs	OVM	>90%	G1 from #372: 58% G1 from #376: 48%	No.	Cas9	Plasmid	Transfection al.,2016	Oishi et
PKFs	CMAH, GTAI	-	0.5%**(double KO)	N.D.	Cas9	mRNA	Sequential SCNTs of edited cell lines	Fischer et al., 2016
			HDR (homology-directed repair)					
BEFs	POLLED introgre-ssion	-	7% (Day 70)	No	TALEN	mRNA, Oligo DNA	SCNT of edited cell lines	Carlson et al., 2016
GFFs	hLF inser -tion after BLG KO	-	40% (3 mo)	N.D.	TALEN	mRNA, pBLG-hLK -puro	SCNT of edited cell lines	Cui et al., 2015

*Genetically modified embroyos per injection zygote (%). ** Genetically modified offspring per injection embryo (%). N.D. : PKF : Porcine Kideny Fibroblast. PGC : Primordial Germ Cell GFF : Goat Fetal Fibroblast. Bovine Embryo Fibroblast. SCNT : Somatic Cell Nuclear Transfer.

Conclusion

Rapid advances in livestock genome editing research suggest that animal products will enter the market soon after their food safety is confirmed in a country. However, previous controversy over GM animals and animal cloning underscores the importance of people's sense of ethics as well as animal welfare.

The breeding of farm animals using genome editing should be performed after due considerations in relation to the ethical implications of animal genetic modification in society. Moreover, for animal welfare, developers should thoroughly investigate the occurrence of off-target mutations in the breeding of genome-edited animals. Regulators should interrogate developers about off-target mutations and promote public dialogues about livestock breeding using genome editing if they wish to enhance the public acceptance without any major disputes in society. Such farm animal products will never be accepted without consideration about both the practical and ethical aspects of animal genome editing.

References

On Request

Chapter 4

Pharmacogenetics : Recent Update in Customization of Therapy

NRIP KISHORE PANKAJ, MUDASIR SULTANA, P.K.VERMA AND RAJINDER RAINA

Div. of Veterinary Pharmacology and Toxicology, F. V. Sc. & A.H., SKUAST-J, R. S. Pura, Jammu, J&K

We often observe that some of the population responses to a conventional therapy and other not, in addition, it may result in to toxicity in some, this happens due to involvement of genetics. This aspect of drugs is dealt under Pharmacogenetics. Therefore it can be stated as "the study of the genetic basis for variation in drug response". Albeit, the term 'Pharmacogenetics' came in to existence in consequence to the Watson and Crick model of DNA in 1953, and coined by Friedrich Vogel in 1959. It has made a significant stride since 2003, but it is yet far from expectations. A vast number of discoveries relating to genomic variability and drug response have been made in the last 10 years.

There is an inter-individuals difference of 300-1000 nucleotides, which estimates a total of 10 million single nucleotide polymorphisms (SNPs; single base pair substitutions). These SNPs are found in the tune of ≥ 1% in a population, and thus thousands copy of a number of variations in the genome (International HapMap *et al.*, 2007). This implies huge numbers of variations along with their combinations. These variations results in to inter individual difference in drug effects. Genetic testing has various implications that includes prediction for treatment related to toxicity or facilitates for dose adjustment, along with determination of adequate response or lack thereof. It must be done before treatment, as giving inappropriate therapy may result in poorer outcome than expected and "treat-and-watch" approach has ethical and legal perspective (Beaulieu *et al.*, 2010). Therefore, it can be said that we are moving towards customization of therapy, and or prevention of ailments before it could become obvious. This implies assessment of multigenic determinants for drug responses. This task is big, lying over the shoulder of modern pharmacogenetics.

Genetic Variations in Pharmacotherapy

Pharmacogenomics is another closely entwined term to pharmacogenetics, which involve tools to survey entire genome. Pharmacogenomic approaches involve efforts to pin point specific inherited variations in order to predict individual subjects' response to therapy. Inherited genetic variation affects the expressions of protein as well as its amino acid sequence. This includes nucleotide repeats, insertions, deletions, translocations and SNPs.

Any polymorphisms in CyP450 family (Aquilante *et al.*, 2004) multidrugs transporters-1 (Panczyk *et al.*, 2009) and other molecular targets, lead to altered expression thereby changed coding and thus activity of the proteins with regard to function changes in phenotype. This includes few clinically relevant examples of genetic defects illustrating the relevance of pharmacogenomics in optimizing treatment, as a way to enhance efficacy and safety. Current anticancer drugs are more specific and focused, have broader therapeutic window with lesser adverse drug action as compared to earlier chemotherapies. New drugs are designed to impede specific molecular target, usually a protein with a critical role in tumor growth or progression (i.e. tyrosine kinase). Such targeted therapies are available which includes monoclonal antibodies, antisense inhibitors, and of tyrosine kinase inhibitors. Most of these agents put selective pressure for cancer cells. Similarly, it appears to happen for protein kinase inhibitor. The best understanding of this problem at a molecular level comes from studies on imatinib resistance in Chronic Myelogeneous Leukaemia (CML) patients carrying BCR/ABL fusion gene. These imatinib-resistant clones, consisting a single nucleotide mutation in ABL Kinase domain (with consequent amino acid substitution), are successfully suppressed by second-generation Tyrosine kinase inhibitors (i.e. Dasatinib, Nilotinib), still active on almost all imatinib-resistant mutants (Bui *et al.*, 2010). Similarly to imatinib, other Gefitinib and Erlotinib have exhibited clinical activity in a subset of patients affected by Non Small Cell Lung Cancer. Gefitinib and Erlotinib are the selective kinase activity inhibitor of epidermal growth factor receptor (Gazdar, 2010). Recently, it has been reported that specific point mutation of epidermal growth factor receptor (EGFR) gene in tumor cells select EGFR mutated patients (Gefitinib-responder), from EGFR wild type (non-responders) in Non-Small Cell Lung Cancer subjects (De Mello, 2011). Such biomarkers are useful to predict specific drug resistance.

HapMap Project

The first phase of the International Hapmap project (2003) has lead to revelation of variety of genetic variations within individuals of diverse ethnic groups in 2003 and facilitated a rich data resource to investigate the correlations of variations in the human genome reflected by a huge variety of clinical phenotypes. This has led to diverse SNP arrays, subject to patient genotype analysis for huge number of SNPs at one time. Further, it aided to pioneer unbiased genetic analysis of clinical phenotype to genotype correlation using platforms created for the Genome Wide Association Study (GWAS). The important factors determining inter-individual variability in drug response, the role of rare, or private, variants is unclear in pharmacogenomics phenotypes, and is an important area for research.

Genomes Project

This genomes project facilitated the scientific community with a population scale map of rare variants to complement and enrich existing knowledge of common variants gained from the HapMap project. This will facilitate studies regarding role of rare genetic variants in defining variation in drug response phenotypes. Mapping of rare and common variants within 12 CyP450 genes has been performed which is thought to be responsible for metabolizing 75% of drugs (Gordon *et al.*, 2014) New and potentially deleterious allele in major drug metabolizing enzymes has been identified among 7.6%–11.7% African Americans and Caucasians. The next generation sequence technologies is used to identify rare variants that can facilitate better understanding of inter-individual variability in drug responses, where common variants explain a limited degree of variability *i.e.* variability is the case of warfarin dose prediction. When CYP2C9*2, *3 and VKORC1 polymorphisms is incorporated, allows clinicians to predict up to 60% (Wadelius, *et al.*, 2009) of dose variability. In future, incorporating the rare functional genetic variants may allow for even greater accuracy in warfarin dose prediction. Rare missense variants have been observed in the VKORC1 gene in warfarin resistant patients (Ainle, *et al.*, 2008; Harrington, *et al.*, 2008). Likewise, drug-induced torsades de point may be due to rare mutations in the congenital long QT syndrome genes (Behr *et al.*, 2013) About 23% of Caucasians carry a variant within 22 congenital arrhythmia genes, including 13 congenital long QT syndrome genes with drug-induced torsades de pointes, compared with a background rate of 1.7% in 60 control subjects from the 1000 Genomes CEU data (Ramirez *et al.*, 2013).

Non-Coding RNAs

The myth of junk DNA in human genome is now unfounded. The presence of non-coding RNAs has altered the perception of the central dogma of molecular biology. The application of small non-coding RNA molecules as biomarkers of variable drug response has been recorded. However, studies have shown the potential utility for specific microRNAs as markers of both drug-induced liver injuries (miR-122 and -192) (Consortium, *et al.*, 2012) and severe skin reactions (miR-18a-5p) (Ichihara *et al.*, 2013). Albeit, such biomarkers are still at the discovery stage, further clinical validation may see these and other non-coding RNAs enter clinical practice as early-stage pharmacogenomics predictors of adverse drug reactions.

Genotyping

Genotyping methods are of two types based on the capability to screen new mutations or identification of known mutations. As such genotyping needs to detect both wild and mutant type of alternate alleles and distinguish between alternative alleles in a DNA sample. There is only one platform which is capable to fulfill both of these tasks in a single step assay is the "Matrix-Assisted Laser Desorption/ Ionization Time of Flight" (MALDI TOF). This platform can involve single tube/phase or "homogeneous reaction" and may involve both phase *i.e.* a liquid and a solid phase called heterogeneous reaction (DNA Chip). The most commonly used platform to detect known SNPs can be:

i) Homogeneous platform.

ii) Heterogeneous platform.

iii) The advantages of homogeneous methods.

iv) Reduced risk of cross-contamination.

v) Time effectiveness and.

vi) Feasibility.

Homogeneous Methods

Conventional methods for SNPs detection *i.e.* Single-Strand Conformational Polymorphism (SSCP) and Restriction Fragment Length Polymorphism (RFLP) are now obsolete and replaced by high-throughput methods. High-throughput processing is feasible now with the aid of robotic processor like 1G Genetic analyzer by Illumina/ Solexa (Cambridge, UK), SOLiD by Applied Biosystems (Foster City, CA, USA) and Genome Sequencer FLX by Roche Diagnostics (Brandfort, CT, USA) using 96 or 384 well plate. These ultra quick DNA sequencers have great accuracy of 99.99%. In contrast to PCR based methods, Non-PCR methods *i.e.* Ligase chain reaction, Rolling Circle Amplification (RCA) and Invader® assays (Third Wave Technologies, Madison, WI, USA) are used to genotype straight way from genomic DNA.

Heterogeneous Methods

It includes methods, such as DNA chip based microarray, Golden Gate® assay and mass spectrometry genotyping technologies. These are the latest development in the genotyping but these are costly affair thus less widely used than cheaper PCR-based methods in the clinical laboratory setting. In addition, to the costs for DNA chip, its interpretation depends on well-trained and qualified personnel. Some of the **common laboratory methods** in pharmacogenomics studies are for **detection and screening for unknown mutations:**

i) Detection and screening.

ii) Conventional sequencing.

iii) Denaturing-HPLC.

iv) Denaturing gradient gel electrophoresis (DGGE).

v) Heteroduplex DNA assay (melting curve).

vi) High throughput sequencing.

vii) Single strand conformation polymorphism (SSCP).

Methods for Detection of Known Mutations

i) Homogenous

a) Fluorescent probe by Allelic Discrimination (Hyb Probe®, TaqMan®, Beacons® Scorpions®) High Resolution Melting (HRM).

b) Invader® assay Locked Nucleic Acid (LNA) probe.

c) Peptide nucleic acid-mediated Clamping PCR.

d) Pyrosequencing.

ii) Heterogenous

a) Gene Chip technology.

b) Golden Gate® assay.

c) Maldi-TOF Mass Spectroscopy.

d) Oligo ligation assay (SNPlex®).

Most significant known genetic variants and their effect in pharmacotherapy

GENE	Polymorphism (nucleotide translation)	Molecular effects	Drug	Effects on therapy
CyP450 family	Variety of polymorphism	Enzyme activity ↓	Many	Inter-individual variability in pharmacokinetics
Thiopurine methyl transferase 2, 3A, 3C	Variety of polymorphism	Enzyme activity ↑	6-mercaptopurine & Thioguanine	Hemopoietic toxicity
UDP-glucuronosyl transferase 1A 28	TA repeats in 5′ promoter	Enzyme activity ↓	Irinotecan	Neutropenia
Multidrug resistance 1	(C3435T)	Low expression	Many	Multiple drug resistance
Thymidylate synthase	3 tandem repeats	Enzymeactivity ↑	5-fluorouracil, Methotrexate	Drug resistance
DPYD	IVS14+1G	Enzyme activity ↓	5-fluorouracil, Methotrexate	Neutropenia
Dihydrofolate reductase	T91C	Enzyme activity ↑	Methotrexate	Drug resistance
5,10-methylene tetra hydrofolate reductase	(C677T) (A1298C)	Enzyme activity ↓	5-fluorouracil, Methotrexate	Toxicity
c-KIT	D860 N567K	Constitutive signal activation	Imatinib	desensitizes activity in GIST
K-RAS	G12x G13D	Inhibition of the tyrosine kinase domainbinding drug	Cetuximab, Panitumomab	Desensitizes activity in colon-rectum carcinoma
B-RAF	V600E	Inhibition of the tyrosinekinase domainbinding drug	Vemurafenib Gefitinib	Good response in melanomas Good response in Non-Small Cell Lung Cancer
Epidermal Growth Factor Receptor	L858R	Inhibition of the tyrosine kinase domainbinding drug	Erlotinib	
BCR/ABL fusion gene	t(9;22) BCR/ABL	Constitutive signal activation	Imatinib, Dasatinib Nilotinib	Good response in Chronic Myeloid Leukemia

ABL	T315I, M351T	Inhibition of the tyrosine kinase domainbinding drug	Imatinib	Drug resistance in Chronic Myeloid Leukemia
PML/RARa fusion gene	(15;17) PML/RARa t	Block of myeloid lineage cells	All Trans Retinoic acid	Good response in Acute Myeloid Leukemia-M3 subtypes cells
adrenergic b receptors B1,B2	R389GG	Altered Gprotein	beta-blockers	Gets desensitized
MHC class B 1	Several SNPs including codon K751Q	HLA-B~5701aplotype	Abacavir	Hypersensitivity
Vitamin K epoxide reductase complex 1	Many, VKORC1 haplotypes codon G3673	Associated with a higher/low Warfarin dose	warfarin	Variable anticoagulant effect

The technology depends on type of mutation, acquired genetic change, or the analysis of inherited SNPs. This explains heterogeneity of sample source. Such sample may contain many wild type DNA. It is thus imperative to have precise and sensible techniques to detect mutant genome of cancer among the backdrop of normal DNA. There are several methods suitable for genotyping to probe for SNPs and or detect mutant allele either in hetero or homozygols cells (Di Francia *et al.*, 2010).

Clinical Utilization of Pharmacogenomics

According to an estimate, over 150,000 studies claimed biomarkers; less than 100 has made it into clinical utility (Poste, 2011) which included pharmacogenomic as well as other biomarkers. There are currently 121 Food and Drug Administation (FDA) drug labels refer to pharmacogenetic biomarkers of drug safety or efficacy (US FDA, 2013). Only a very small proportion of these drug labels mandate clinicians to test for pharmacogenetic markers (e.g., abacavir and HLA-B*57:01; and carbamazepine and HLA-B*15:02 in Southern Asians). Many pharmacogenetic biomarkers have failed to move from discovery to clinical implementation especially in relation to adverse drug reactions. These include drug-induced skin injury (Pirmohamed *et al.*, 2011), liver injury (Pirmohamed *et al.*, 2011a) and Torsade de Pointes (Behr *et al.*,, 2012).

Genetic Biomarkers of Adverse Drug Reactions

SNP alleles rs4149056 (c.521T>C/*5), associated to loci SLCO1B1 in Caucasian produce myopathy with the drug Simvastatin, that is commonly used to treat hypercholesterolaemia in other population

(Link *et al.*, 2008). SNP alleles rs1934951, associated to loci CYP2C8 among Spanish population causes Osteonecrosis of the jaw with the drug Bisphosphonate indicated for multiple myeloma (Sarasquete *et al.*, 2008). Caucasian population do possess SNP *07 and *02, associated to HLA-DRB1 loci results in to hepatotoxicity on administration of an anticoagulant Ximelagatran (Kindmark *et al.*, 2008). HLA-B loci associated to SNP B*57:01 among Caucasian, when treated with antibiotic flucloxacillin leads to hepatotoxicity (Daly *et al.*, 2009). Japanese Causasian with HLA-A loci associated SNP A*31:01 exhibit skin rash and or hypersensitivity with cabamazepine indicated for epilepsy (McCormack *et al.*, 2011; Ozeki *et al.*, 2011).

Ethical Issue

The implementation of customized medicine may relate to the health inequalities, within and between countries. The costs factor related to developing, manufacturing and getting approval for genetic tests, in addition to defining the role of ethnic genetic differences, it would be tough for resource poor countries to get benefits of customized medicine advances in the future.

Another issue is with the use of next generation sequencing technologies, whether patients should be informed about incidental findings.

Regulatory Environment

There are regulatory concerns which need to be tackled in order to facilitate the implementation of pharmacogenomic testing into clinical practice. The regulatory environment has a big influence on the diagnostics industry as well. With the development of companion diagnostics, it will be vital so as to streamline procedures which facilitate approval of the drug and diagnostic. There are differences between the FDA and European Medicines Agency, with the latter being less stringent, but likely to adopt similar procedures in a drive to ensure there is global harmonization of the regulatory procedures needed for approval (Senderowicz and Pfaff, 2014).

The Future

The polymerase chain reaction was pioneered by Kary Mullis in 1983 (Saiki, *et al.*, 1988), facilitated sensitive analysis of DNA and led to a number of pharmacogenetic biomarkers in the pre-genome era.

The PCR-based technology has advanced significantly and allows for rapid and accurate genotype detection. Pre-treatment genetic testing guides for drugs used are anticoagulant coumarin derivatives (e.g., warfarin) (Pirmohamed *et al.*, 2013) and the antiplatelet drug clopidogrel (Roberts *et al.*, 2012). In warfarin trial, it was found that patients randomized to pharmacogenetic-guided dosing, spent a mean percentage time in the therapeutic range of 67.4% compared with 60.3% on the standard dosing protocol (Pirmohamed *et al.*, 2013). In the case of the RAPID-GENE trial (Roberts *et al.*, 2012), patients were typed for the CYP2C19*2 allele, which has been associated with a lack of efficacy of clopidogrel following percutaneous coronary intervention (PCI). This study demonstrated that genotype-guided dosing significantly reduced adverse events (platelet reactivity) compared to standard treatment. The genotyping technology utilized for RAPID-GENE, the Spartan RX CYP2C19, is able to produce genotypes in less than 60 min. POC Genotype technologies continue to advance and molecular biology methodologies, such as SmartAmp 2 (Lezhava *et al.*, 2010) are reducing the time to obtain a genotype further. It is already possible to determine genotypes for pharmacogenomics-related variants, such as those associated with warfarin dose requirement (VKORC1 and CYP2C9) in 30–40 min (Lezhava *et al.*, 2010; Aomori *et al.*, 2009). With addition of microfluidics technology to devices (Burn, 2013; Stedtfeld *et al.*, 2012), the size of the equipment for genotyping decreases and subsequently, enhance portability. In future years, it is likely that many more advanced devices and tests would be applied to clinical care and obtain regulatory approval.

References

Ainle, F.N.; Mumford, A.; Tallon, E.; McCarthy, D.; Murphy, K. A vitamin k epoxide reductase complex subunit 1 mutation in an Irish patient with warfarin resistance. Irish J. Med. Sci. 2008, 177: 159–161.

Aomori, T.; Yamamoto, K.; Oguchi-Katayama, A.; Kawai, Y.; Ishidao, T.; Mitani, Y.; Kogo, Y.; Lezhava, A.; Fujita, Y.; Obayashi, K.; et al., Rapid single-nucleotide polymorphism detection of cytochrome p450 (cyp2c9) and vitamin k epoxide reductase (vkorc1) genes for the warfarin dose adjustment by the smart-amplification process version 2. Clin.Chem.2009, 55: 804-812.

Aquilante CL, Lobmeyer MT, Langaee TY, Johnson JA. Comparison of cytochrome P450 2C9 genotyping methods and implications for the clinical laboratory. Pharmacotherapy 2004; 24: 720-726.

Beaulieu M, De Denus S, Lachaine J. Systematic review of pharmacoeconomic studies of pharmacogenomic tests. Pharmacogenomics 2010; 11: 1573-1590.

Behr, E.R.; January, C.; Schulze-Bahr, E.; Grace, A.A.; Kaab, S.; Fiszman, M.; Gathers, S.; Buckman, S.; Youssef, A.; Pirmohammed, M.; et al., The international serious adverse events consortium (isaec) phenotype standardization project for drug-induced torsades de pointes. Eur. Heart J. 2012. 34: 1958–1963.

Behr, E.R.; Roden, D. Drug-induced arrhythmia: Pharmacogenomic prescribing? Eur. Heart J. 2013, 34: 89–95.

Bui MR, Hodson V, King T, Leopold D, Dai S, Fiolkoski V, Oakes S, Duke R, Apelian D, Franzusoff A, Degregori J. Mutation-specific control of BCRABL T315I positive leukemia with a recombinant yeast-based therapeutic vaccine in a murine model. Vaccine 2010; 28: 6028-6035.

Burn, J. Company profile: Quantumdx group limited. Pharmacogenomics 2013, 14: 1011–1015.

Consortium, E.P.; Bernstein, B.E.; Birney, E.; Dunham, I.; Green, E.D.; Gunter, C.; Snyder, M. An integrated encyclopedia of DNA elements in the human genome. Nature 2012, 489: 57–74.

De Mello RA, Marques DS, Medeiros R, Araujo AM. Epidermal growth factor receptor and K-Ras in non-small cell lung cancer-molecular pathways involved and targeted therapies. World J Clin Oncol 2011; 2: 367-376.

Di Francia R, Frigeri F, B Erretta M, Cecchin E, Orlando C, Pinto A, Pinzani P. Decision criteria for rational selection of homogeneous genotyping platforms for pharmacogenomics testing in clinical diagnostics. Clin Chem Lab Med 2010; 48: 447-459.

Gazdar AF. Tyrosine kinase inhibitors and epidermal growth factor receptor (EGFR) mutation in non-small cell lung cancer: to test or not to test? Medicine (Baltimore) 2010; 90: 168-170.

Gordon, A.S.; Tabor, H.K.; Johnson, A.D.; Snively, B.M.; Assimes, T.L.; Auer, P.L.; Ioannidis, J.P.; Peters, U.; Robinson, J.G.; Sucheston, L.E.; et al., Quantifying rare, deleterious variation in 12 human cytochrome p450 drug-metabolism genes in a large-scale exome dataset. Hum. Mol. Gen. 2014. 23: 1957–1963

Harrington, D.J.; Gorska, R.; Wheeler, R.; Davidson, S.; Murden, S.; Morse, C.; Shearer, M.J.; Mumford, A.D. Pharmacodynamic resistance to warfarin is associated with nucleotide substitutions in vkorc1. J. Thrombosis Haemost. 2008, 6: 1663–1670.

Ichihara, A.; Wang, Z.; Jinnin, M.; Izuno, Y.; Shimozono, N.; Yamane, K.; Fujisawa, A.; Moriya, C.; Fukushima, S.; Inoue, Y.; et al., Upregulation of mir-18a-5p contributes to epidermal necrolysis in severe drug eruptions. J. Allergy Clin. Immunol. 2013, 133: 1065–1074.

International HapMap Consortium. The international hapmap project. Nature 2003, 426: 789–796.

Kindmark, A.; Jawaid, A.; Harbron, C.G.; Barratt, B.J.; Bengtsson, O.F.; Andersson, T.B.; Carlsson, S.; Cederbrant, K.E.; Gibson, N.J.; Armstrong, M.; et al., Genome-wide pharmacogenetic investigation of a hepatic adverse event without clinical signs of immunopathology suggests an underlying immune pathogenesis. Pharmacogenomics J. 2008, 8: 186–195.

Lezhava, A.; Ishidao, T.; Ishizu, Y.; Naito, K.; Hanami, T.; Katayama, A.; Kogo, Y.; Soma, T.; Ikeda, S.; Murakami, K.; et al., Exciton primer-mediated snp detection in smartamp2 reactions. Hum. Mut. 2010, 31: 208–217.

Link, E.; Parish, S.; Armitage, J.; Bowman, L.; Heath, S.; Matsuda, F.; Gut, I.; Lathrop, M.; Collins, R. Slco1b1 variants and statin-induced myopathy—A genomewide study. New Engl. J. Med. 2008, 359: 789–799.

McCormack, M.; Alfirevic, A.; Bourgeois, S.; Farrell, J.J.; Kasperaviciute, D.; Carrington, M.; Sills, G.J.; Marson, T.; Jia, X.; de Bakker, P.I.; et al., Hla-a*3101 and carbamazepine-induced hypersensitivity reactions in europeans. New Engl. J. Med. 2011, 364: 1134–1143.

Ozeki, T.; Mushiroda, T.; Yowang, A.; Takahashi, A.; Kubo, M.; Shirakata, Y.; Ikezawa, Z.; Iijima, M.; Shiohara, T.; Hashimoto, K.; et al., Genome-wide association study identifies hla-a*3101 allele as a genetic risk factor for carbamazepine-induced cutaneous adverse drug reactions in japanese population. Hum. Mol. Gen. 2011, 20: 1034–1041

Panczyk M, Balcerczak E, Piaskowski S, Jamroziak K, Pasz-Walczak G, Mirowski M. ABCB1 gene polymorphisms and haplotype analysis in colorectal cancer. Int J Colorectal Dis 2009; 24: 895-905.

Pirmohamed, M.; Aithal, G.P.; Behr, E.; Daly, A.; Roden, D. The phenotype standardization project: Improving pharmacogenetic studies of serious adverse drug reactions. Clin. Pharmacol. Ther. 2011, 89: 784–785.

Pirmohamed, M.; Burnside, G.; Eriksson, N.; Jorgensen, A.L.; Toh, C.H.; Nicholson, T.; Kesteven, P.; Christersson, C.; Wahlstrom, B.; Stafberg, C.; et al., A randomized trial of genotype-guided dosing of warfarin. New Engl. J. Med. 2013, 369: 2294–2303.

Pirmohamed, M.; Friedmann, P.S.; Molokhia, M.; Loke, Y.K.; Smith, C.; Phillips, E.; La Grenade, L.; Carleton, B.; Papaluca-Amati, M.; Demoly, P.; et al., Phenotype standardization for immune-mediated drug-induced skin injury. Clin. Pharmacol. Ther. 2011, 89: 896–901.

Poste, G. Bring on the biomarkers. Nature 2011, 469: 156–157.

Ramirez, A.H.; Shaffer, C.M.; Delaney, J.T.; Sexton, D.P.; Levy, S.E.; Rieder, M.J.; Nickerson, D.A.; George, A.L., Jr.; Roden, D.M. Novel rare variants in congenital cardiac arrhythmia genes are frequent in drug-induced torsades de pointes. Pharmacogenomics J. 2013, 13: 325–329.

Roberts, J.D.; Wells, G.A.; Le May, M.R.; Labinaz, M.; Glover, C.; Froeschl, M.; Dick, A.; Marquis, J.F.; O'Brien, E.; Goncalves, S.; et al., Point-of-care genetic testing for personalisation of antiplatelet treatment (rapid gene): A prospective, randomised, proof-of-concept trial. Lancet 2012, 379: 1705–1711.

Saiki, R.K.; Gelfand, D.H.; Stoffel, S.; Scharf, S.J.; Higuchi, R.; Horn, G.T.; Mullis, K.B.; Erlich, H.A. Primer-directed enzymatic amplification of DNA with a thermostable DNA polymerase. Science 1988, 239: 487–491.

Sarasquete, M.E.; Garcia-Sanz, R.; Marin, L.; Alcoceba, M.; Chillon, M.C.; Balanzategui, A.; Santamaria, C.; Rosinol, L.; de la Rubia, J.; Hernandez, M.T.; et al., Bisphosphonate-related osteonecrosis of the jaw is associated with polymorphisms of the cytochrome p450 cyp2c8 in multiple myeloma: A genome-wide single nucleotide polymorphism analysis. Blood 2008, 112: 2709–271

Senderowicz, A.M.; Pfaff, O. Similarities and differences in the oncology drug approval process between fda and european union with emphasis on in vitro companion diagnostics. Clin. Cancer Res. 2014, 20: 1445–1452.

Stedtfeld, R.D.; Tourlousse, D.M.; Seyrig, G.; Stedtfeld, T.M.; Kronlein, M.; Price, S.; Ahmad, F.; Gulari, E.; Tiedje, J.M.; Hashsham, S.A. Gene-z: A device for point of care genetic testing using a smartphone. Lab. Chip 2012, 12: 1454–1462.

US Food and Drug Administration. Table of Pharmacogenomic Biomarkers in Drug Labeling. Available online: http://www.fda.gov/drugs/science research/researchareas/pharmacogenetics/ucm083378.htm/ (2013).

Wadelius, M.; Chen, L.Y.; Lindh, J.D.; Eriksson, N.; Ghori, M.J.; Bumpstead, S.; Holm, L.; McGinnis, R.; Rane, A.; Deloukas, P. The largest prospective warfarin-treated cohort supports genetic forecasting. Blood 2009, 113: 784–792.

□□□

Chapter 5

Chromatographic and Spectrometric Techniques in Monitoring Quality Control of Foods of Livestock Origin

ARVIND KUMAR*, SAKSHI SHARMA*
NEELESH SHARMA AND ATUL ANAND****

* Division of Livestock Products Technology, F.V.Sc & A.H., SKUAST-Jammu
** Division of Veterinary Medicine, F.V.Sc & A.H., SKUAST-Jammu

Introduction

The development of new methods that might or might not involve sophisticated techniques for the quality control of food products continues increasing according to consumer requirement of food safety and authenticity issues. The production of fakes is a worldwide problem that includes food products. Some examples can be found on olive oils, honeys and alcoholic beverages, such as table wines and spirits .Therefore, food authentication concerns both authorities and food processors to avoid the unfair competition from counterfeiters who exploited the economic advantage by producing and selling fake food products. Food companies have adopted different strategies to improve the positioning of their brands on the market. These strategies not only include the food quality control based on the identification and reduction of forbidden compounds but also on monitoring the key compounds that enhance the food value. In this chapter a practical review of methods for quality control on compounds and on the confirmation of food authenticity is presented. Non-destructive testing sample methodologies that have found new applications in the field of quality assurance are discussed in terms of their potential use in food industry. The optimization of the analytical methods is based on the selection of fundamental working conditions (sampling, pretreatment, selectivity, linearity, range determination, sensitivity, limit of detection, precision and accuracy, etc.) according to which the suitability of a selected method might be evaluated. One of the most important steps in the analytical method for compound determination in biological matrices is the sample pretreatment. The purpose of a pretreatment is to release analytes from compounds and phases as well as to remove components, which have adverse impacts on the analytical signal (Contreras *et al.*, 2010).

Chromatographic Techniques

It has been widely used because they offer good information about sample composition. Their principal advantages are separation efficiency; identification of almost any type of molecule present in a food sample; and depending of which technique is employed, it is possible to obtain very low detection limits for a wide range of analytes. Liquid chromatography, in particular HPLC (*high performance liquid chromatography*), can detect compounds, such as aldehydes, proteins, amino acids, phenolic compounds and carbohydrates (Schultheiss *et al.*, 2000). On the other hand, G C (*gas chromatography*) is more suited to the analysis of volatile or semi-volatile compounds; some substances must be extracted from the food sample, e.g., fatty acids from triglycerides; but others, such as alcohols, can be injected directly into the column. The most commonly detectors used for chromatographic techniques involve UV-Vis (*ultraviolet–visible*), fluorescence, electrochemical, MS (*mass spectroscopy*), FID (*flame ionization detector*), ECD (*electron capture detector*), electronic nose, etc. The methods developed through these techniques have established patterns of composition of several types of samples by monitoring the specific compounds. The principal disadvantage of chromatographic techniques is the complex operation which requires special training to ensure that the technique is performed correctly. False results are obtained when the laboratory equipment involved with the technique is not operated correctly. Besides, long analysis times are required (Petroviæ *et al.*, 2010).

Gas Chromatography

Basically, chromatograph equipment consists of four systems: gas supply, the sampling, the column and the detector system. The gas supply system provides, depending on the kind of detector that is chosen, the necessary type of gas or gas mixture. The sampling system usually contains an automatic injector that is situated inside a thermostatically controlled enclosure and generally has its own oven, but sometimes shares the column oven for temperature control. The injector can have a complex transport system that can take samples, wash containers, prepare derivatives and, if necessary, carry out a very complex series of sample preparation procedures before injecting the sample onto the column. The column is the principal device that actually achieved the necessary separation, and has an oven to control the column temperature. Finally, for detection there is a wide range of detectors available, each having unique operating parameters and its own performance characteristics. The best selection depends on the sample nature and this system also has its own oven. The analyzed substances through GC must be volatile and should be vaporized and moved through a long column by an inert carrier gas. The column is filled with a packing material covered with a not-volatile liquid. The molecules of each substance will be distributed into the gas and the liquid. The more volatile a substance is the longer it will be moving with the carrier gas, and the quicker it will emerge from the column. The sample pretreatment usually is complex and the compounds of importance, usually, must be extracted from the matrix but if they are not volatile then derivatization techniques must be used. The extraction of an analyte utilizes the partitioning of a material between two phases and it is based on solubility or insolubility in various solvents. Extraction is useful for sample preparation and purification, but is also often a first step in qualitative analysis. There are several kinds of extraction process, such as liquid-solid, liquid-liquid, SPE (*solid phase extraction*) and SPME (*solid-phase micro-extraction*) (García *et al.*, 2011).

In liquid-solid extraction, a solvent (hydrophilic or hydrophobic, acidic, neutral or basic) is added to a solid. Insoluble material can be separated by gravity or vacuum filtration, and soluble material is extracted into the solvent. A sequence of solvents, by varying polarity or pH, can be used to separate complex mixtures into groups. Then, the filtered solution can be injected into the GC system. If the two phases are immiscible liquids the technique is called liquid-liquid extraction. Usually, one phase is aqueous (hydrophilic) and the other is a hydrophobic organic solvent. A sequence of extractions with more than one solvent can be used to separate, with considerable efficiency, relatively complex mixtures. SPE uses the affinity of solutes dissolved or suspended in a liquid (known as the mobile phase) for a solid through which the sample is passed (known as the stationary phase) to separate a mixture into desired and undesired components. The result is that either the desired analytes of interest or undesired impurities in the sample are retained on the stationary phase. The portion that passes through the stationary phase is collected or discarded, depending on whether it contains the desired analytes or undesired impurities. If the retained portion on the stationary phase includes the desired analytes, they can then be removed from the stationary phase for collection in an additional step in which the stationary phase is rinsed with an appropriate eluent. SPME involves the use of a fiber coated with an extracting phase, that can be a liquid (polymer) or a solid (sorbent), which extracts different kinds of analytes (including both, volatile and non-volatile) from different kinds of media that can be in liquid or gas phase. The amount of extracted analyte by the fiber is proportional to its concentration in the sample as long as equilibrium is reached. Then, the fibre is transferred to the injection port of the gas chromatograph where desorption and analysis of the analytes is carried out (Gilbert *et al.*, 2010).

The most typical applications on GC for food analysis pertain to the quantitative and/or qualitative analysis of food composition, natural products, food additives, flavour and aroma components; a variety of transformation products, and contaminants, such as pesticides, fumigants, environmental pollutants, natural toxins, veterinary drugs, and packaging. Among the natural products analyzed by GC one can highlight the analysis on olive oil samples. Recent studies are based on the determination of several kinds of analytes such as undesirable compounds, e.g. pesticides and herbicides (Aramendía *et al.*, 2007); monoaromatic volatile compounds (benzene, toluene and ethylbenzene); beneficial health compounds such as phenolic compounds (García and Aparicio, 2007); studies that involve the interpretation of the responsible compounds of oil aroma (Garcia Gonzalez & Aparicio, 2010) and so on. There are other works that analyze changes of patterns focused on comparison of their fatty acid composition through chemometric analysis. Chemometric analysis of the triacylglycerol and fatty acid composition is usually a media to determine their varietal and geographical authenticity (Luykx and van Ruth, 2008). GC offers good information about distillated beverages composition and its utility has been proved on the analysis of spirit beverages like tequila, vodka, cognac, rum and brandy. Through a variety of detectors, such as FID, MS, electronic nose, etc., coupled to GC equipment it has been possible to establish patterns of composition and concentration not only for white but for rested alcoholic beverages (aged in barrels) too. For these beverages aldehydes, phenols, terpenes, higher alcohols, volatile organic acids, esters, fatty acids, etc. are monitored (Plutowska and Wardencki, 2008).

HPLC

HPLC is a separation technique that involves the injection of a small volume of liquid sample into a tube packed with tiny particles (3 to 5 ìm in diameter). Individual components of the sample are moved down the packed tube (column) with a liquid (mobile phase) forced through the column by high pressure delivered by a pump. For the case of LC (*liquid chromatography*), samples are transported along the column by a liquid moved by gravity.

In principle, LC and HPLC work in similar way but HPLC has some advantages over LC such as speed, efficiency, sensitivity and ease of operation, and they make it vastly superior to LC. The compounds in a sample are separated one from the other by the column packing that involves various chemical and/or physical interactions among their molecules and the packing particles. These separated components are identified at the exit of the column by a flow-through device (detector) that measures them. The detector device can be based on several techniques, such as a spectrophotometric, fluorescence or electrochemical detection. The output from the detector is called a chromatogram. The HPLC equipment is constituted by four principal components, i.e. the pump, the injector, the column and the detector systems [10].

The pump system forces a liquid (mobile phase) through the column at a specific flow rate and normal flow rates in HPLC are in the range of 1-to 2-mL/min. Typical pumps can reach pressures in the range of 6000-9000 psi (400-to 600-bar). During the chromatographic experiment a pump can deliver a constant mobile phase composition (isocratic) or an increasing mobile phase composition (gradient).

The injector serves to introduce the liquid sample into the flow stream of the mobile phase. Typical sample volumes are 5-to 20-microliters (ìL) and the injector must also be able to withstand the high pressures of the liquid system. When the user has many samples to analyze or when manual injection is not practical, then the use of an autosampler is recommended (this is an automatic version).

The column system is considered the "heart of the chromatograph". The column's

Stationary phase separates the sample components of interest using various physical and chemical parameters. The pump must push hard to move the mobile phase through the column and this resistance causes a high pressure within the chromatograph. It is important to take into account that the correct selection of the column packing and the mobile phase are the most important factors in making the best performance with HPLC.

The detector can determine individual molecules that come out (elute) from the column. A detector serves to measure the amount of those molecules so that the chemist can quantitatively analyze the sample components. The detector provides an output to a recorder called chromatogram.

To separate most compounds there are four major separation modes, i.e. RPC (*Reversed-Phase Chromatography*), Normal Phase or Adsorption Chromatography, Ion Exchange Chromatography and SEC (*Size Exclusion Chromatography*).

For RPC the column packing is non-polar, e.g. C18, C8, C3, phenyl, etc. and the mobile phase is water (buffer) + water-miscible organic solvent, methanol and acetonitrile. RPC is by far the most popular mode (over 90%) and can be used for non-polar, polar, ionizable and ionic molecules. All this makes to RPC very versatile for samples containing a wide range of compounds; gradient elution is often used. One begins with a predominantly water-based mobile phase and then adds organic solvent as a function of time. The organic solvent increases the solvent strength and elutes compounds that are very strongly retained on the RPC packing.

The Normal Phase technique or Adsorption Chromatography is useful for water-sensitive compounds, geometric isomers, cis-trans isomers, class separations, and chiral compounds. The column packing is polar (e.g. silica gel, cyanopropyl-bonded, amino-bonded, etc.) and the mobile phase is non-polar (e.g. hexane, iso-octane, methylene chloride, ethyl acetate), normal phase separations are performed less than 10% of the time. Ion Exchange Chromatography, in this mode the column packing contains ionic groups, e.g. sulfonic, tetraalkylammonium and the mobile phase is an aqueous buffer, for example phosphate or formate. Ion exchange is used for about 20% of the cases and it is well suited for the separation of inorganic and organic anions and cations in aqueous solution, Ionic dyes, amino acids, and proteins. In fact any salt compounds in brine water. In size exclusion chromatography, there is no interaction between the sample compounds and the column packing material. Instead, molecules diffuse into pores within a porous medium and depending on their size (relative to the pore size) molecules can be separated. Thus, molecules larger than the pore opening do not diffuse while those smaller do and get separated. Large molecules elute first while smaller molecules elute later. The SEC technique is used by 10-15% of the cases, mainly for polymer characterization and for proteins.

Modern agriculture and food processing often involve the use of chemicals. Some of these chemicals and their functions are listed below:

- Fertilizers: increase production of agricultural plants
- Pesticides: protect crops against weeds and pests
- Antibiotics: prevent bacteria growth in animals during breeding
- Hormones: accelerate animal growth
- Colorants: increase acceptability and appeal of food
- Preservatives and antioxidants: extend product life
- Natural and artificial sweeteners and flavors: improve the taste of food
- Natural and synthetic vitamins: increase the nutritive value of food
- Carbohydrates: act as food binders.

Electronic nose

Electronic nose technology is based on chemical gas-sensor array technology, i.e. the detection by an array of semi-selective gas sensors of the volatile compounds present in the headspace of a food sample. Some of the advantages of the electronic nose technology over other techniques are the high number of samples that can be analyzed in a short period of time, with good reproducibility and accuracy. However, this technique employs sensors that are not very selective for particular types of compounds, thus, preventing any real identification or quantization of individual compounds present in a food sample. Electronic nose technology in conjunction with chemometric analysis has also been successfully applied to the analysis of changes of aroma, along days, released from a flavour encapsulated in a polysaccharide gel matrix, i.e. the time dependence of the aroma pattern emitted by an encapsulated essence. Chemometric analysis is also applied to alcoholic beverages, such as wine samples. Spanish white, red and rose wines were differentiated using a combination of electronic nose and principal components analysis. On the other hand, authenticity studies have also been carried out for the differentiation of honey samples. Other applications include the determination of the geographical origins of food products and the differentiation of olive oils from adulterated samples with other kind of oils. Despite its drawbacks, electronic nose technology remains an area of research that holds much potential for future development in a higher number of applications related to food. Numerous electronic nose studies related to food already have been published. Many of them represent preliminary feasibility studies, but a limited number of them represent basic studies including long term validation of the technique on a specific application [11].

Spectroscopic Techniques and Chemometric Tools

Spectroscopic techniques have the potential to simplify and reduce analytical times. This section reviews the use of some spectroscopic techniques, which combined with chemometric assess food quality. Among the techniques that will be considered are Raman, NIR, MIR, NMR, UV-Vis and fluorescence. Some of the main advantages of spectroscopic methods are simplicity, rapidity, and practically there is no use of sample pre-treatment. However, the capacity of simultaneous determination of several analytes in the same sample or the determination of a single analyte in complex matrices through direct spectroscopic measures diminishes because the spectral overlap. Chemometric tools such as the MVCM (*multivariate calibration models*) allow the spectral resolution and quantification in the presence of interferents. The advantage of using data involving high-dimensional structured information is the higher stability towards interferents and matrix effects compared with first-order methodologies. There are several algorithms for analyzing second-order data, such as PARAFAC, BLLS (*bilinear least-squares*) and N-PLS (*multiway partial least*-squares) [12].

The Raman, Mid-infrared (MIR 4000 to 400 cm^{-1}) and Near-infrared (NIR 14000 - 4000cm^{-1}) spectroscopic techniques

The use of Raman, MIR and NIR spectroscopic techniques in chemical analysis has been broadened for the past two decades due to the advance of technological and scientific innovations. The involved instrumentation in these three techniques is easy to implement at any laboratory, for academic or industrial use, due to the increase of improved instruments in the market. Furthermore, for routine processes these techniques are very practical since special training is not required and the cost of the equipment would be much less than any of those use in chemical analysis. The main feature of these techniques when applied to any sample is that they are not destructive and the time to obtain results is short compared to wet analysis. Thus, if they are applied to food products for quality control the sample under study does not require any pre-treatment. When Raman spectroscopy is compared against IR spectroscopy, it presents the advantage of low sensitivity to water; therefore lends itself for making measurements in liquid environments. On the other hand, it presents high sensitivity to C=C, Ca"C and Ca"N bonds and thus, the fatty acid composition in foods is easily determinate. Raman spectroscopy also gives high selectivity to inorganic compounds like salts. The Raman spectroscopy has been employed for determination of food proteins. For this case, Raman spectra of modified proteins trough analysis of a new C=O stretching vibrational band attributed to -carboxyl groups of aspartic and glutamic acids was used. For quantitative measurements of carotenoid, collagen and fat in fish muscle, the Raman technique was also used. In the case of edible oil analysis, the Raman technique allowed to investigate the chemical changes taking place during lipid oxidation in several edible oils through oxidative degradation of several vegetable oils by using heating at 160°C [13].

NMR Spectroscopy

NMR spectroscopy involves the analysis of the energy absorption by atomic nuclei with non-zero spins in the presence of a magnetic field. The energy absorptions of the atomic nuclei are affected by the nuclei of surrounding molecules, which cause small local modifications to the external magnetic field. NMR spectroscopy can therefore provide detailed information about the molecular structure of a food sample, given that the observed interactions of an individual atomic nucleus are dependent on the atoms surrounding it. High-resolution NMR (HR-NMR; frequencies above 100 MHz) has been applied in many food products. NMR is conventionally used to obtain detailed chemical information on liquid-state systems. Recent advances in techniques and hardware now allow the routine acquisition of high-resolution ^{13}C NMR spectra from solid materials [14].

Fluorescence and UV–Vis Spectroscopy

Fluorescence spectroscopy has been used to assess different food proprieties by using different methods, such as synchronous front-face fluorescence spectroscopy along chemometric methods. Fluorescence spectroscopy can determinate some properties of food products without sample preparation, since it is a non-destructive technique; there is no use of chemicals; food can be solid or liquid and the time of performance to obtain results can be very short, when compared against those wet techniques; it can be used to analyze compounds at concentration as low as parts per billion, and among anything many food products contain intrinsic compounds that emit light, when excited with the proper light-wavelength [15].

Conclusions

In addition to sensory parameters such as aroma, colour or taste, the quality of food all over the world is based on measurable factors, such as chemical and nutritional composition (percentage of sugar, fatty acids, antioxidants, protein, fibre etc.), as well as microbiological control. In this chapter, an over view of some of the most used methodologies for quality control of food products has been shown. It is clear that chemical analysis plays an important role in this matter and the choice of appropriate analytical method should be treated as an essential aspect. This is so since the chosen method for analysis should be adequate to the purpose for which results are required, e.g., determination of forbidden and permitted substances (application of food laws and official regulations) or monitoring of key compounds that enhance the food value. Besides the suitable method of analysis, it was pointed out in this chapter that sampling and pre-treatment of food products play an important rule in the quality control process for food products. A short review of sampling procedures was given and the pre-treatment on food was pointed out along the presented analytical method.

New trends on the quality control processes are clearly seen now-a-days. Industry needs to reduce costs and time during the test of food products. Besides high levels of specificity and accuracy, analysis along the line of production is needed. Pre-treatment of samples should be minimized to reduce costs and times for testing food products. Thus, in this chapter it was shown that there are a great variety of analytical methods for food quality control. However, those based on chromatography are the best bet since new methodologies with chemometric analysis are rising up. The main developments in chromatographic methods are focused on the reductions of analysis times.

References

1. Contreras, U., Barbosa Garcia, O., Pichardo Molina, J.L., Ramos Ortiz, G., Maldonado Rivera, J.L., Meneses Nava, M.A., Ornelas Soto, N.E., López-de-Alba, P.L. (2010). Screening method for identification of adulterate and fake tequilas by using UV–VIS spectroscopy and chemometrics. *Food Research nternational*, Volume 43, Issue 10, December 2010, pp. 2356-2362.

2. Schultheiss, J., Jensen, D., Galensa, R. (2000). Determiantion of aldehydes in food by highperformance liquid chromatography with biosensor coupling and micromembrane suppressors. *Journal of Chromatography A*, Volume 880, Issues 1-2, 2 June 2000, pp. 233-242.

3. Petroviæ, M., Keziæ, N., Bolanèa, V. (2010). Optimization of the GC method for routine analysis of the fatty acid profile in several food samples. Food *Chemistry*, Volume 122, Issue 1, 1 September 2010, pp. 285-291.

4. García Villalba, R., Pacchiarotta, T., Carrasco Pancorbo, A., Segura Carretero, A., Fernández Gutierrz, A., Deelder, A.M., Mayboroda, O.A. (2011). Gas chromatography– atmospheric pressure chemical ionization-time of flight mass spectrometry for profiling of phenolic compounds in extra virgin olive oil. *Journal of ChromatographyA*, Volume 1218, Issue 7, 18 February 2011, pp. 959-971.

5. Gilbert Lopez, B., Robles Molina, J., García Reyes, J., Molina Diaz, A. (2010). Rapid determination of BTEXS in olives and olive oil by headspace-gas chromatography/mass spectrometry (HS-GC-MS). *Talanta*, Volume 83, Issue 2, 15 December 2010, pp. 391-99.

6. Aramendía, M.A., Borau, V., Lafont, F., Marinas, A., Marinas, J.M., Moreno, J.M., Urbano, F.J., (2007). Determination of herbicide residues in olive oil by gas chromatography–tandem mass spectrometry. *Food Chemistry*, Volume 105, Issue 2, 2007, pp. 855-861.

7. García Gonzalez, D.L., Aparicio, R. (2010). Coupling MOS sensors and gas chromatography to interpret the sensor responses to complex food aroma: Application to virgin olive oil. *Food Chemistry*, Volume 120, Issue 2, 15 May 2010, pp. 572-579.

8. Luykx, D., van Ruth, S. (2008). An overview of analytical methods for determining the geographical origin of food products. *Food Chemistry*, Volume 107, Issue 2, 15 March 2008, pp. 897-911.

9. Plutowska, B., Wardencki, W. (2008). Application of gas chromatography–olfactometry (GC–O) in analysis and quality assessment of alcoholic beverages- A review. *Food Chemistry*, Volume 107, Issue 1, 1 March 2008, pp. 449-463.

10. González Rodriguez, R.M., Rial Otero, R., Cancho Grande, B., Simal Gandara, J. (2008). Determination of 23 pesticide residues in leafy vegetables using gas chromatography–ion trap mass spectrometry and analyte protectants. *Journal of Chromatography A*, Volumes 1196-1197, 4 July 2008, pp. 100-109.

11. Rodríguez, M., Durán, I., Ornelas, N., López de Alba, P.L., López L., (2008). Determination of anticarcinogenic and rescue therapy drugs in urine by photoinduced spectrofluorimetry using multivariate calibration: comparison of several secondorder methods. *Anal. Bioanal. Chem.*, 391 (2008) pp. 1119-1127.

12. Rodriguez, S.D., Monge, M.E., Olivieri, A.C., Negri, R.M., Bernik, D.L., (2010). Time dependence of the aroma pattern emitted by an encapsulated essence studied by means of electronic noses and Chemometric analysis. *Food Research International*, Volume 43, Issue 3, April 2010, pp. 797-804.

13. Muik, B., Lendl, B., Molina-Díaz, A., Ayora-Cañada, M.J., (2005). Direct monitoring of lipid oxidation in edibl e oils by Fourier transform Raman spectroscopy. *Chemistry and Physics of Lipids*, Volume 134, Issue 2, April 2005, pp. 173-182.

14. Consonni, R., Cagliani, L.R., (2010). Nuclear Magnetic Resonance and Chemometrics to Assess Geographical Origin and Quality of Traditional Food Products. *Advances in Food and Nutrition Research*, Volume 59, 2010, Chapter 4, pp. 87-165.

15. Mattarucchi, E., Stocchero, M., Moreno-Rojas, J., Giordano, G., Reniero, F., and Guillou, C., (2010). Authentication of Trappist Beers by LC-MS Fingerprints and Multivariate Data Analysis. *J. Agric. Food Chem.*, 58 (23), 2010, pp. 12089–12095.

□□□

Chapter 6

Prospects for Viral Disease Control with Plasmid DNA Vaccines in Veterinary Practice

RAJESH AGRAWAL AND NISHI PANDE*

Division of Veterinary Medicine
* Division of Veterinary Gyanecology and Obsterics
F.V.Sc & A.H., SKUAST-J, R.S. Pura- 181 102

Vaccines are one of the most cost-effective disease control technologies. Traditional vaccines have many practical disadvantages regarding their production, usage and efficacy (Meeusen *et al.,* 2007). Gene-based vaccination offers an attractive alternative to traditional vaccine strategies (Nguyen *et al.,* 2008). The protein targets of immune responses, termed antigens, are encoded in DNA and produced within the body's own cells, which can mimic live infection more closely than injection of traditional non-replicating vaccines (Gurunathan *et al.,* 2000). Intracellular production of antigens from DNA can result in co-ordinated activation of both humoral and cell-mediated responses.

The property of naked DNA to get transfected to mammalian cells in vivo was first reported by Ito (1960); and three decades later, the concept of DNA vaccine was evolved by Wolff *et al.* (1990), when they administered a recombinant bacterial plasmid DNA to obtain the expression of â-galactosidase gene in mice. This paved way for the development of nucleic acid based vaccination, an effective way for the *in vivo* expression of desired protein to initiate immune response (Oshop *et al.,* 2002 and Liu, 2003). The application of DNA immunization as a new generation vaccine has undergone clinical trials for many viral diseases, in veterinary practice like foot and mouth disease (FMD) and herpes virus infection in cattle, Aujeszky's disease and classical swine fever in swine, rabies and canine distemper in canines, and avian influenza, infectious bronchitis and infectious bursal disease in birds (Dhama *et al.,* 2008).

Essential features of a DNA vaccine construct

DNA vaccines, generated using plasmids, include a gene encoding target antigen under the transcriptional control of an effective viral/ eukaryotic promoter, along with a poly-adenylation signal sequence (poly-A) and a bacterial origin of replication (Gurunathan *et al., 2000*). The commonly used promoter has been derived from cytomegalovirus (CMV). The poly-A provides stability and effective translation, where the antibiotic resistance gene facilitates selection of bacteria. For complete optimization, the plasmid should have Kozak sequence (GCCA/GCC) upstream of initiator codon, and an enhancer, downstream of the poly-A signal (Fig. 1).

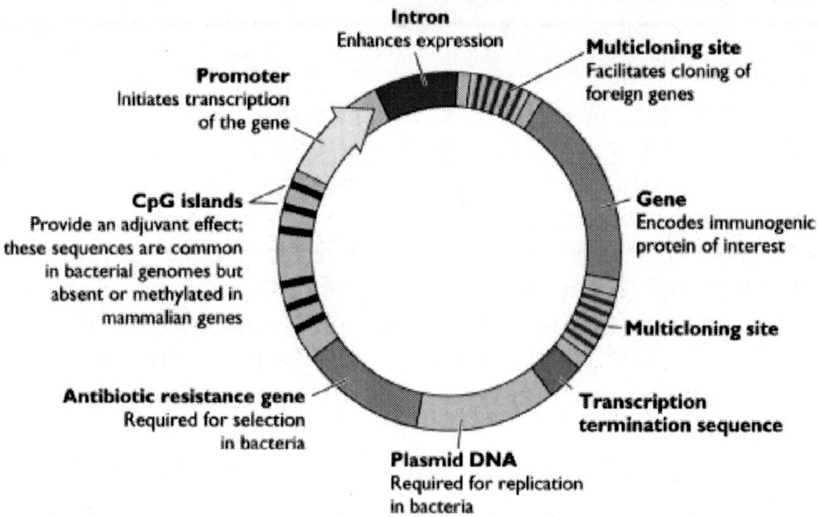

Fig. 1. Diagrammatic representation showing essential features of a DNA vaccine construct.

DNA vaccine in comparison with other conventional vaccine

DNA vaccines stimulate the MHC I pathway of the immune system, the major effector cells of which are CD8 suppressor T lymphocytes. DNA vaccines heighten cell mediated immunity. Conventional vaccines stimulate humoral immunity and the production of soluble antibodies (immunoglobulins) through MHC II pathway. Conventional vaccines use as an antigen either live attenuted or killed microorganism, or purified protein from the coat of the organism. DNA vaccines achieve MHC I responses by presenting the antigen intracellularly. In fact, vaccination by DNA fragments shot into muscle by gene gun produces both MHC I and MHC II responses of varying degrees of intensity. The major need for DNA vaccine is to stimulate cellular rather than humoral immunity. Table 1 summarizes the differences between conventional and DNA vaccination (Ross, 2002 and Rawat *et al.*, 2007).

Table 1. Differences between Conventional and DNA vaccination

Issues	Conventional Vaccination	DNA Vaccination
Immune response	Antibody	Antibody and T-cell
Complete antigen repertoire	x	✓
Duration of response	Variable	Long
Number of required vaccine dose	Multiple	One or more
Safety (especially pregnant and immunosuppressed individuls)	Unsafe	Safe
Risk of reversion	✓	X
Impaired efficacy in the presence of maternal antibodies	✓	X
Ease of production	Difficult	Easy
Cost	Expensive	Inexpensive
Cold storage	Required	Not required
DIVA (Differentiating Infected from Vaccinated Animals)	x	✓

Mechanism of action of DNA vaccines

The mechanism of immune induction by which genetic vaccines confer protection still remains unclear. The slow rise of the immune response following DNA immunization suggests that it follows a complex pathway that can mimic natural viral infection. However, it is believed that once the DNA plasmid is administered to the skin, subcutaneum, vein, nasal cavity or muscle, the plasmid vector enters the cell, translocates to the nucleus and the transcription of the immunogene is initiated using the host's cellular machinery. The two major types of cells that become transfected through this method are myocytes and antigen-presenting cells (APCs). Following transfection, the host cell's replication machinery translates the transgene into protein, the peptides of which are subsequently presented by MHCI to the immune system. Additionally, antigenic protein can be secreted in and around the surrounding tissue either by active secretion of the protein or its release following apoptosis of a transfected cell. The shed antigenic protein can then be engulfed and presented by APCs on both, MHC-I and MHC-II, after which, the antigen-loaded APCs can migrate to the corresponding draining lymph node to activate naive T cells. Costimulatory signals help to trigger an immune response and the recruitment of more T cells (Kutzler and Weiner, 2008). At the lymph node, the T cells' secreted cytokines and shed antigens activate B cells and induce antibody production. The initial wave of T- and B-cell activation is small, but once these cells migrate back to the vaccine-transfected tissue, they can undergo restimulation. At this point, CD8+ T cells can lyse transfected myocytes presenting antigenic peptide on their MHC-I molecules, causing the release of more antigen. Furthermore, CD4+ T cells can activate immature dendritic cells (DCs) that later drain to the lymph node and take on a whole new cohort of B and T cells (Reyes-Sandoval and Ertl, 2001), repeating the cycle of activation again. Therefore, both, humoral and cellular immune responses are primed for their next challenge.

Innate immunity: Antigen expression alone is not enough to induce efficient immune responses. The body does not normally activate immune responses against "self" antigens and generally requires a "danger signal" to discriminate between "foreign" and "self" antigens.

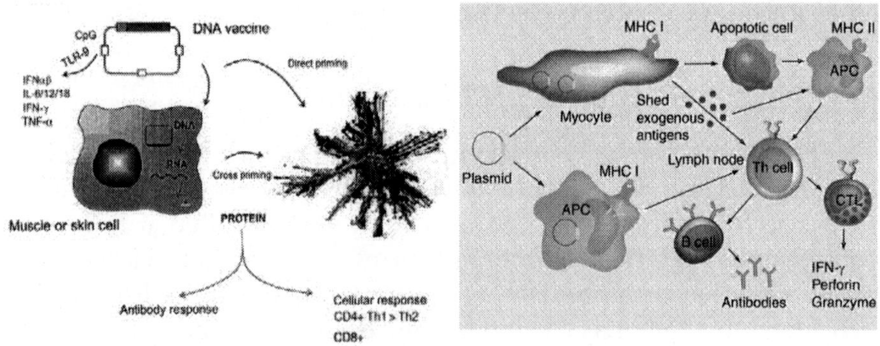

Fig. 2. Pathways of cell-mediated and humoral immune responses to DNA vacciness

Thus, supplying a second danger signal is equally as important as achieving efficient antigen expression. APCs express PRRs that recognize structurally and evolutionarily conserved motifs on bacteria or viruses. During infection, these PRRs provide the secondary danger signal early (minutes to hours) prior to the generation of an adaptive immune response (Akira *et al.*, 2006). Danger signals can also include chemicals released by damaged cells, stimuli from other immune cells or interaction with foreign materials.

Factors determining the immunogenicity of DNA vaccines

The various factors along with remarks (Wolfgang *et al.*, 1999) have been presented in Table 2.

Table 2. Factors determining the immunogenicity of DNA vacciness

Factors	Remarks
Structure of the plasmid backbone	Presence of immunostimulatory sequences, introns, poly-A-sequence
Amount of plasmid delivered	More is better
Expression levels of the antigen	More antigen correlates with stronger response, but not necessarily linearly
Immunization schedule	Increasing interval between immunizations can strongly enhance the response
Route of immunization	Intramuscular, intradermal (needle), epidermal (gene gun), mucosal
Target-tissue	Including what muscle is injected or what section of the skin
Number of immunizations	DNA-induced immune response can effectively be boosted with DNA
Presence or absence of introns in front of the gene	Introns increase efficacy
Strain of the particular species	Different mouse strains show qualitative and quantitative differences in DNA-induced immune responses
Age of animals	Stronger response the younger the mice
Toxicity of the antigen for transfected host cell	High expression undesirable for toxic antigens

The Different Mechanical and Physical Techniques of Administration

a) Needle injection

Direct injection of DNA solution into a tissue to achieve gene transfer was reported by Wolff *et al.* in 1990 using plasmid containing a reporter gene. With needle injection a solution of plasmids is delivered typically into muscle or skin, subcutaneously or intradermally. The solubility and the volume of the vaccine is a limiting factor of where and how precise the injection can be performed, which means that for instance an epidermal needle injection is technically difficult. The most widely employed delivery method is intramuscular injection; naked DNA in saline is injected directly into skeletal muscle tissue using a hypodermic needle. The induced immune response is primarily a TH1 cell-mediated immune response (Sin *et al.*, 1999). Liu *et al.* (1999) reported that a rapid injection of a large volume of DNA solution via the tail vein of a mouse led to highly efficient gene delivery to hepatocytes. Hagstrom *et al.* (2004) showed that highly efficient gene transfer into muscle tissue in dogs and primates can be achieved by a procedure involving injection of plasmid DNA into a distal vein of a limb that is transiently isolated by a tourniquet or blood pressure cuff.

b) Intralymphatic injection

Recently, it has been shown that administration of DNA directly into lymph nodes, described as intralymphatic immunotherapy (ILIT), induces powerful immune responses. Intralymphatic DNA administration has been found to be safer and 100- to 1000-fold more effective in the generation of cytotoxic T lymphocyte responses than intramuscular DNA delivery, and to generate high titre antibody responses consistent with a T helper-1 response (Senti *et al.*, 2009, Martinez-Gomez *et al.*, 2009). Intralymphatic vaccination has also been successfully introduced to veterinary field. In a pilot study low dose DNA vaccination into submandibular lymph nodes of ponies using plasmid expressing the equine influenza virus haemagglutinin successfully led to seroconversion with IgG antibody titres comparable to current commercial protein based equine influenza vaccines (Landolt *et al.*, 2010).

c) Gene gun or particle bombardment

A gene-gun is a device for administration of plasmid coated on microscopical gold-particles. The gold-particles adhere to the inside of a plastic tube and they are blown out by high-pressure helium and driven into the tissue. Thereby plasmids can be delivered directly into the cytoplasm of the cells in the epidermis, including Langerhans cells (Pertmer *et al.*, 1996). Particles are "shot" into the cells of the skin, so the extracellular barrier is removed. Significantly lower amounts of

DNA are needed by this technique. For large animals, sites may be chosen with little hair, for example, around the tail and auxillary regions of the legs. The animals do not show any discomfort. Helios gene gun system from Bio-Rad Laboratories uses a helium discharge to deliver gold particles. The gene gun may also be used to vaccinate cows intravulvomucosally. The major limitations of the current gene gun technology are dose limitation (approximately 1 ìg in each shot), difficulty to prepare uniform microparticles, and limited access to target cells deep in the tissue.

d) Needle-Free Injection /Biojector

The development of needle-free injection originally stemmed from a general apprehension of needle injections, disease transmission by accidental needle-sticks, and the need for effective mass immunization. Several different jet injectors have been used to deliver DNA vaccines in cattle against bovine respiratory syncytial virus (Schrijver *et al.*, 1998) and in pig for pesudorabies DNA vaccine (van Rooij *et al.*, 1998). It has been shown to improve efficacy of DNA vaccines as compared with needle injection because of better distribution of the plasmid in the target tissue, which may be skin or muscle. This then may result in large numbers of cells being transfected. In addition, although not entirely painless, needle-free delivery devices avoid potential tissue damage in food-producing animals. A number of needle-free devices are available, including the Biojector 2000, the Pigjet™ injector (van Rooij *et al.*, 1998) and the Injex 30 Needle Free Injector System. The Biojector 2000 used for DNA immunization of pigs, sheep, and cattle consists of an injection device, a disposable needle-free syringe, and a CO2 cartridge, which can deliver between 10 and 15 injections with proper technique. A tank adapter for a large CO2 tank is available for the Biojector 2000 System. Biojector is a registered trademark for another needleless device for administration of DNA vaccines. It shoots an ultra-fine stream of plasmid-containing liquid into the tissue by means of high pressure. It can be targeted to inject volumes upto 1 ml intramuscularly, subcutaneously and intradermally.

e) Topical/ Tattooing

Topical administration to skin of a DNA-vaccine has been done successfully. Merely painting the DNA-vaccine on intact skin did produce an immune response. A technique, which removes the keratinocytes and reveals the germinative layers of the skin, for instance, by ripping them off with aid of a fast-acting adhesive, showed better result. This is followed by application of a saline solution of plasmid-DNA to the newly exposed skin and both humoral and cell mediated immune response to the vaccine antigen was shown (Liu *et al.*, 2001). It has been proven that topical delivery of plasmid DNA with suitable adjuvants to the skin of the chicken (wing web region) results in a wide distribution of the plasmid with protein production in several tissues.

f) Electroporation

Currently, one of the most effective techniques for administration of plasmids DNA is electroporation. The principle behind electroporation is to temporarily permeabilize cell membranes to allow for increased uptake of large molecules, such as plasmid DNA. It is more effective in enhancing the level of expression in muscle tissue compared to skin tissue (Babiuk *et al.*, 2003). Electroporation causes cellular infiltration into the electroporated tissue, which is important in generating an immune response following DNA immunization (Babiuk *et al.*, 2004). It works effectively in several animal species like rat, rabbit, pig, sheep, goat, cattle and monkey; different types of electrodes currently in use, like needle-free patch, single-needle and multipleneedle array electrodes (Babiuk *et al.*, 2006). The skin is an ideal tissue to use needle-free patches, whereas the muscle in larger animals requires the more invasive needle electrodes to be effective. It is important that electroporation parameters should be optimized for each animal species, because tissues, such as skin vary dramatically between species with respect to thickness as well as lipid composition. Two different types of EP protocols have been developed. First uses only low voltage (LV) electric pulses with long duration (100-200 V/cm, 20-50 ms). In the second, a combination of one high voltage (HV) electric pulse (600-800 V/cm, 100 ìs) followed by different numbers of LV electric pulses (80-100 V/cm, duration in time range of tens to hundreds of milliseconds) is used (Satkauskas *et al.*,2005). Pavlin *et al.* (2008) showed that combination of 1 high voltage pulse (600 V/cm, 100 ìs), followed by 4 low voltage pulses (80 V/cm, 100 ms, 1 Hz) yielded in the same transfection efficiency as the standard trains of low voltage pulses. The results indicate that electrotransfection is a feasible, effective, and safe method for muscle targeted gene therapy in dogs, which could have potential for clinical applications in veterinary medicine of small animals.

g) Suppositories

Scientists developed a simpler method to vaccinate cows mucosally by formulating the plasmid in suppositories. These suppositories can be delivered intravaginally with ease and produce subsequent protective immune responses to intranasal challenge to bovine herpesvirus-1 (BHVI) (Loehr *et al.*, 2001). It was the first report of mucosal immunity by non-invasive DNA immunization against bovine herpesvirus-1, where cows were immunized intravaginally with suppositories containing plasmid coding for glycoprotein D. Serum IgG, as well as IgA both in the serum and in the nasal fluids, were detected, which supports the contention of a common mucosal immune system. This level of immunity was of sufficient magnitude to minimize weight loss and significantly reduce the duration of virus shedding after intranasal viral challenge, which demonstrates the efficacy of suppository-based administration of DNA vaccines to target species. As this is a very practical method of delivery, it has great potential to be applied as vaccine or therapy in a variety of species.

Synthetic particles as DNA vaccines delivery systems

There exists a clear need for new vaccine delivery systems that can be administered at low doses to elicit strong humoral and cellular immune responses. Synthetic particles may prove to be a drastic improvement for the current generation of naked DNA vaccines, which have a low transfection efficiency and immunogenicity. One promising approach is the development of microparticles and nanoparticles as delivery systems for DNA vaccines (Cui and Mumper, 2003).

Particulate vaccine delivery systems can induce cytotoxic T lymphocyte (CTL) - and other cell-mediated immunity to key pathogens including viral infections. DNA delivery can be achieved by gold-coated particles, liposomes, inert macro-, microspheres and nano-beads. Inert particles coated or conjugated to antigen are designed to provide a targeted immune response. Encapsulation of antigen has been widely used for its easy delivery, slow release and protection from degradation of the antigen with an effective single dose. Nanoparticles range from 10 to 500 nm, while microparticles are larger, around 1–100 ìm in diameter. Solid particles are made from inert materials or biodegradable polymers. Biodegradable and biocompatible polyesters, such as polylactide-co-glycolides (PLG) have been extensively used to encapsulate antigens.

Advantages of particles

The majority of particle formulations use electrostatic interaction between anionic phosphate groups in DNA with a cationic carrier, usually composed of building blocks with positively charged nitrogen atoms. In this complex formation process, an excess of carrier DNA is condensed into positively charged, nano-sized particles is advantageous (in contrast to naked DNA) for vaccination in that it confers protection against endonuclease-mediated degradation upon injection (Goh *et al.*, 2004) and has the potential to increase cellular uptake of nucleic acids, which can lead to higher transfection efficiencies. Smaller particles (<100 nm) have a much higher transfection activity than larger particles. The upper size limit of particles that can be taken up by non-phagocytotic cells is approximately 500 nm (Gaumet *et al.*, 2009). To further increase cellular uptake of particles, cell- penetrating peptides (CPPs) can be coupled to the particle surface (Vives *et al.*, 2008). Uptake by antigen presenting cells is strongly dependent on both, particle size and surface charge of the particles. Larger particles, with a size between 0.5 and 5 ìm can be specifically taken up by APCs via phagocytosis. DNA containing particles can also activate immature APCs, which lead to an increased expression of co-stimulatory molecules and release of cytokines. This up-regulation can be beneficial for vaccine formulations and depends on the characteristics of the particles used.

a) Lipid-Based Gene Carriers

Cationic lipids are the oldest (Felgner *et al.*, 1987) and most commonly used delivery vehicles for genetic vaccines. In general, these cationic lipids with so-called helper lipids are formulated into unilamellar liposomes before they are complexed with DNA. Upon electrostatic interaction of a cationic liposome with negatively charged DNA, nano-sized complexes are formed, called lipoplexes. Lipoplex delivery of DNA probably works through a combination of a potent adjuvant effect. The presence of the lipid provides the plasmids with enhanced stability in the GIT and also, some protection against degradation by nucleases *in vivo*. Lipoplexing as a delivery strategy therefore, has potential to improve antigen delivery to antigen presenting cells (APCs). Gene delivery efficiency of lipoplexes is influenced primarily by lipid structure, charge ratio, the environment, where gene delivery is carried out, and the type of cells employed. Commonly used cationic lipids are, 1,2-dioleoyl-3-trimethylammonium

(DOTAP), which is used most frequently as the gold standard in lipid DNA carriers and L-alpha-dioleoyl phosphatidylethanolamine (DOPE) or cholesterol to increase the transfection properties of the DNA/lipid complexes (Christensen *et al.*, 2007). A major obstacle for the wider use of these carriers in gene therapy is their toxicity, which is due to the cationic nitrogen group in these molecules (Lappalainen *et al.*, 1994).

b) Cationic polymer Based Gene Carriers

Cationic polymers are widely used as delivery vehicles for genes in both in vitro and in vivo applications (De Smedt *et al.*, 2000). Electrostatic complexation of a cationic polymer with negatively charged DNA results in a nanoparticle called a polyplex. The major advantages of polymers above lipids upon complexation with genes are that particle sizes are generally smaller and the polymer structure can be easily modified to tailor the characteristics of the formed particles. The two classical polymers used for gene transfer applications are poly (ethylenimine) (PEI) and poly (l-lysine) (PLL). Cationic polymers generally show higher toxicity than the lipds (Roques *et al.*, 2009), which is positively correlated to the molecular weight of the polymer. Another disadvantage of polymers is their lower biodegradability compared to lipids. Degradation of the polymeric carrier can also be used to increase the release of DNA from the polyplex in the cytosol (Funhoff *et al.*, 2004).

c) Micro-/Nano-particles Based Gene Carriers

Although cationic compounds are most commonly used, non-ionic polymers are also useful as a vehicle for DNA vaccine delivery. Poly lactide (PLA) or poly lactide-co-glycolide (PLGA) is most commonly used since these polymers are biodegradable and non-toxic. PLGA particles can be produced in the micro to nanoscale size range. DNA can be encapsulated inside these particles using different techniques such as spray-drying or solvent evaporation (Jilek *et al.*, 2005). Another strategy is to adsorb DNA onto the surface of these particles after coating with a cationic compound such as PEI or cetyltrimethylammonium bromide (CTAB). The advantage of adsorption is that the plasmid is not exposed to the acid microenvironment that is formed inside the particles upon degradation of PLGA particles. A disadvantage of adsorption is that the loading efficiency upon adsorption is lower than the already low efficiency upon encapsulation (max ~1% of particle mass). Protection against nuclease degradation has been demonstrated for both, encapsulated and adsorbed DNA (Oster *et al.,* 2005). Another possible advantage of micro-sized carrier systems is that due to their size, they are preferentially taken up by APCs upon *in vivo* administration (Newman *et al.,* 2002). A major hurdle is that uptake should be followed by expression of the antigen-encoding DNA. Several in vitro studies showed that the transfection of DCs is relatively low for these systems (0-10%) (Jilek *et al.,* 2005), especially without the help of physical techniques like electroporation. Microencapsulation of DNA, or association of DNA with microcapsules, has led to enhancement of CTL responses to encoded proteins. It elicits both, CD8+ and CD4+ T cell responses by releasing antigen intracellularly (Doria-Rose and Haigwood, 2003).

The efficacy of orally delivered DNA vaccines has been improved by encapsulating plasmid DNA in PLG microparticles for protection from gastric environment. Experiments carried out with PLG microparticles containing DNA encoding a known CTL epitope of vesicular stomatitis virus (VSV) demonstrated induction of VSV peptide-specific CTL responses (Hedley *et al.,*1998). Thus, nano- and microparticles have the ability to control the release of encapsulated antigen and are safe, suggesting that they may be applied for veterinary vaccines.

Effective dose of DNA vaccine

The dose used in mice depends on the method of administration. Usually an immune response is generated, when 10-100 μg of plasmid DNA is injected IM and 0.1-1 μg, when it is administrated with gene gun (Fynan *et al.,* 1993). Immune response is increased, when 1 or 2 boosters are given (Fuller *et al.,* 1997). Amount of plasmid DNA used for IM inoculation of small animals are 100-300 μg, however, higher doses appear to be required in large animals and humans, with most studies using 0.5-2.5 mg but, while using 'gene gun', only one hundredth of this amount is required (Dunham, *2002*). The difference in dose is applicable to probably reflect the efficiency, by which the plasmid DNA is delivered to the host target cells.

Influence of the route of DNA delivery

a) Gene-gun, intradermal and intramuscular routes of delivery

The efficacy of DNA vaccines varies not only according to the route of delivery, but also to the animal species and pathogen. In chickens, gene gun delivery of DNA vaccine to influenza virus is the most efficient delivery route for DNA immunisation (Fynan *et al.*, 1993). In pigs, i.m. injections of a DNA vaccine against CSFV provided higher levels of antibodies than the gene gun route (Andrew *et al.*, 2000), and intradermal (i.d.) injections of PRV plasmid induced a higher immune response than i.m. injections (van Rooij *et al.*, 1998). In dogs, i.m. injection of a DNA vaccination against rabies virus resulted in a higher and more durable antibody response than that obtained by i.d. injection (Osorio *et al.*, 1999).

b) Delivery of DNA vaccines at mucosal sites

In pigs, DNA vaccination against influenza virus was more effective by g.g. administration on the inferior surface of the tongue than by i.d. injection (Macklin *et al.*, 1998). Intravulvomucosal gene gun vaccination against BHV-1 induced higher humoral and cellular immune responses than vaccination through i.d. injection in cattle (Loehr *et al.*, 2000). Gene-gun administrations at cutaneous and mucosal sites in horses provided a high frequency of seroconversion and total protection against equine influenza virus, whereas cutaneous gene gun administration only induced partial protection (Lunn *et al.*, 1999). All successful mucosal DNA vaccination trials reported to date have used gene gun administration of the vaccine, with the exception of DNA vaccination of chickens against influenza virus (Fynan *et al.*, 1993). Immunisation against influenza virus with DNA drops administered by intratracheal route only provided protection in 30 % of the vaccinated chickens and was less efficient than gene gun delivery.

c) Encapsulation of plasmid DNA into synthetic particles (Liposomes/ Cationic polymers /micro/nano-particle)

Compared to naked DNA that elicits partial protection against BVDV, i.m. vaccination with plasmid DNA encapsulated in cationic liposomes was found to be totally ineffective (Harpin *et al.*, 1999). A DNA vaccine construct containing the VP1 sequence of FMDV serotype O in pVAC vector was formulated by adsorbing plasmid DNA construct on cationic micro particles and administered in guinea pigs @25 µg DNA vaccine construct per animal intramuscularly. It showed enhanced immune response in PLG adjuvanted DNA vaccine. MTT and 3H Thymidine incorporation have shown good CMI responses to PLG adjuvanted DNA (Jadav *et al.*, 2011).

Fate of plasmid DNA after injection

a) Plasmid DNA uptake mechanisms

Before the gene of interest can be expressed, the injected plasmid DNA must overcome three obstacles. The **first obstacle** involves crossing the plasma membrane. DNA is a polyanion and thus, cannot interact with cell plasma membranes, which are negatively charged. There are two main active uptake mechanisms: fluid-phase endocytosis, i.e. not mediated by a receptor and adsorptive endocytosis. Uptake mechanisms depend on certain sequences that may be specific to cell type (Lehmann and Sczakiel, 2005). The **second obstacle** is crossing the cytoplasm. The presence of organelles and the high concentration of proteins in cytoplasm limit the diffusion of large macromolecules, such as plasmid DNA (Luby-Phelps, 2000). The microinjection or electroporation delivery methods have shown that plasmid DNA associates with proteins that resemble dyneins, whereby the microtubule network help transport plasmid DNA to the nucleus (Vaughan and Dean, 2006). Plasmid DNA can also cross the cytoplasm by endocytosis. When endosomes engulf a plasmid, plasmid DNA is protected from degradation for most of its journey to the nucleus. Crossing the nuclear membrane is the **third obstacle**. Plasmid DNA may finally enter the nucleus in two ways: either by taking advantage of nuclear membrane disassembly in dividing cells or by crossing an intact membrane by facilitated diffusion via nuclear pore complexes (NPCs) (Ludtke *et al.,* 2002).

b) Cellular distribution

Dupuis *et al.* (2000) demonstrated that 5 minutes after intramuscular injection with rhodamine-labelled DNA, the DNA was localised in and between myocytes and expresses the gene of interest. It is also present in antigen-presenting cells, such as macrophages and B cells.

c) Tissue distribution

Whatever the route of administration, the site of injection is the area, where the plasmid remains the most concentrated and persist the longest. The mechanism involved in the dissemination of plasmid DNA throughout the body has not been completely determined. However, the presence of plasmids in immune cells (Dupuis *et al.*, 2000), in lymph (Zhang *et al.*, 2005) and blood (Winegar *et al.*,1996) may contribute to their dissemination.

d) Clearance of Plasmid DNA

After intramuscular injection, plasmid DNA is either transfected into cells or it remains free in the body. It is difficult to differentiate between the fate of transfected plasmid DNA and the fate of free plasmid DNA. The clearance of free plasmid DNA may be induced by different factors. The presence of endonucleases in mouse muscle mediated the degradation of 95 to 99% of naked plasmid DNA within 90 min of intramuscular injection, which most likely occurred in the extracellular space (Barry *et al.*, 1999). Zhang *et al.* (2005) showed that higher quantities of plasmid DNA are found in blood than in organs. Some plasmids in the bloodstream may be degraded by nucleases present in blood. Some are eliminated in urine and faeces.

DNA vaccine immune response and protection in neonates

Vaccination of neonates provokes two important questions: Is the neonate's immune system sufficiently mature to elicit a response? Can offspring of an immune mother be immunised despite the high levels of passively transferred maternal antibodies to the antigen?

Three-day-old lambs vaccinated with DNA expressing a gB secreted form of BHV-1 developed both, humoral and cellular immune responses three weeks after vaccination, thereby demonstrating the capacity of the ovine immune system to respond to DNA vaccination at this age. Lambs produced by hyperimmune ewes also responded in the same manner, showing that the maternal antibodies did not prevent development of the anti-BHV-1 immunity in lamb neonates (van Drunen Littel-van den Hurk *et al.*, 1999). In one day old piglets PRV maternal antibodies inhibit the antibody response till 10 or 16 weeks of age, following one or two injections of a gD plasmid. Piglets born from a seronegative sow and vaccinated twice with gD plasmid produced very low levels of neutralising antibodies at 16 weeks. However, these piglets were not protected following subsequent challenge (Monteil *et al.*, 1996).

DNA vaccination was evaluated in chicken neonates against IBDV. Four of seven chicken neonates born, from a non-immune hen produced antibodies after immunisation with a plasmid encoding the polyprotein VP2-VP3-VP4 (Fodor *et al.*, 1999). However, the chickens were not protected against subsequent infection. The injection of a plasmid coding solely for VP2 did not induce an antibody response. Griot *et al.* (2003) demonstrated that despite the presence of maternal antibodies puppies can be vaccinated using the CDV DNA vaccine and that this vaccination has a clear priming effect leading to a solid immune response after a booster with a conventional CDV vaccine.

Enhancing the immunogenicity of DNA vaccines

a) Prime-boost vaccines

Although DNA vaccines have been excellent at inducing protective immune response against some pathogens, particularly in murine models, they have been less potent against other pathogens, and in larger animals. One method that has been used to enhance vaccine efficacy is to combine a DNA vaccine with an alternative immunogen (e.g. protein subunit, killed inactivated microorganism, or viral vector). In the majority of cases, a DNA vaccine is given to prime the immune system, followed by boost using another vaccine; this has generally proven more effective than giving DNA or other type of vaccine followed by a DNA boost (Gurunahan *et al.*, 2000). Liang *et al.* (2006) compared DNA, protein and DNA prime–protein boost regimens against BVDV infection. Groups of calves were immunized with pMASIA-tPAsDE2 or with rDE2, or first with pMASIA-tPAsDE2 and then with rDE2. To evaluate the protection against BVDV, calves were challenged with BVDV strain NY-1 after the last immunization. The DNA prime–protein boost group was stronger than those elicited by either the DNA vaccine or the protein vaccine. In particular, E2-specific antibody titres were enhanced significantly after boosting the DE2 DNA-primed calves with rDE2 protein. There was a significant reduction in weight loss, viral excretion and lymphopenia, compared with the unvaccinated calves and the animals immunized with the DNA or protein only.

b) Co-administration of immunostimulating molecules coding genes

In addition to inducing both, antigen specific cellular and humoral immunity, DNA vaccine technology is able to modulate the amplitude and nature of the immune response through codelivery of plasmids expressing immunostimulating molecules. Genes encoding co-stimulatory molecules involved in antigen binding, such as CD80, CD86 and B7.2, or encoding cytokines involved in the recruitment of antigen presenting cells, such as granulocyte macrophage-colony stimulating factor (GM-CSF) and IL-12 are good candidates for the enhancement of immune responses to viruses (Dufour, 2001). The addition of genes encoding the cytokines GM-CSF, IFN-ã, IL-12, IL-16 and IFN-á to DNA vaccines has been tested in animals. For example, the addition of porcine GM-CSF gene to a DNA vaccine against PRV increased clinical protection in pigs (Somasundaram *et al.*,1999), by enhancing T cell, but not B cell, responses following infection (Dufour *et al.*,2000). The gene coding for IFN-γ was added to a vaccine against feline immunodeficiency virus (FIV) (Hosie and Jarret, 1999) containing the proviral DNA with the *pol* gene deleted. The addition of IFN-ã enhanced clinical protection against FIV, by revealing a decreased viral load after infection compared to cats that had not received IFN-ã. In contrast, the addition of the IFN-ã gene in pigs reduced clinical protection against PRV (Somasundaram *et al.*,1999), as did the addition of the IL-2 (Somasundaram *et al.*,1999) and IFN-á genes (Dufour *et al.*,2000). Addition of feline IL-12 plasmids to a mini-circle2 DNA vaccine against FIV decreased the viral load after infection compared to the same DNA vaccine without IL-12. The IL-12 gene increased CTL activity and reduced FIV seroconversion following challenge (Boretti *et al.,* 2000).

c) Addition of CpG motifs

CpG dinucleotides are unmethylated and present at an expected frequency in bacterial DNA, whereas they are under-represented and selectively methylated in vertebrate genomes (Cardon *et al.,* 1994). Thus, vertebrates recognize bacterial DNA as a pathogen-associated pattern (Krieg *et al.,* 1998). By binding Toll-like receptors, CpG can activate dendritic cells and macrophages to trigger the production of interleukin-1 (IL-1), IL-6, IL-12 and TNF-á as well as natural killer cells and lymphocytes to produce gamma interferon (IFN-γ), IL-6, IL-10 and immunoglobulin, respectively (Hartmann *et al.,* 2000). CpG DNA and CpG oligodeoxynucleotides (ODNs) stimulate Th1-type responses, characterized by IL-12 and IFN-ã secretion with little production of Th2 cytokines and a predominance of IgG2a over IgG1 in the mouse. The high efficacy of CpG ODN as an adjuvant has been demonstrated in a number of species (Ioannou *et al.*, 2002). Petrini *et al.* (2011) indicated that vaccination of calves with a DNA vaccines expressing tgD of BoHV-1 combined with GpG motifs has been able to prime the immune system. However, this response was able to protect animals only partially from virulent BoHV-1 challenge. However, van Drunen Littel-van den Hurk *et al.* (2008) found that the plasmid encoding a secreted truncated version of gD formulated with CpG, effectively primed the immune system of newborn lambs, whereas without CpG the tgD protein was less effective. Furthermore, a heterologous DNA prime-protein/CpG boost induced strong and balanced protective immune responses in newborn calves with BoHV-1-specific maternal antibodies. **Dory** *et al.* (2005) evaluated the adjuvant activity of a porcine-specific type A CpG-containing oligodeoxynucleotide (CpG-ODN) in a DNA-vaccine against Pseudorabies virus (PrV) infection. This vaccine, composed of three independent plasmids encoding PrV gB, gC and gD glycoproteins, was injected alone or was co-injected with CpG-ODN or control GpC-ODN. CpG-ODN improved the PrV-specific humoral and cell-mediated immune response and provided better clinical protection against lethal PrV-infection.

d) Injection of multigenic vaccines

DNA vaccination trials in domestic animals indicate that multigenic injections could be more effective than injections of only one plasmid. Mixtures of plasmids have often been used to obtain protective immunity, either to protect against several viral subtypes, for example, influenza virus (Kodihalli *et al.*, 2000) or to increase protection against a single virus, such as PRV (Dufour *et al.*, 2000, Somasundaram *et al.*, 1999), IBDV (Fodor *et al.*, 1999) or CDV (Cherpillod *et al.*, 2000). A mixture of plasmids coding for several antigens does not always result in protective immunity. This is the case of DNA vaccination against FMDV, for which the injection of three plasmids coding for three viral proteins was not protective in pigs (Beard *et al.*, 1999). Recently, Rao *et al.*, (2009) developed an effective trivalent DNA vaccine that elicits broad protection against different H5N1 sublineages in poultry. It encodes HA proteins from 3 different H5N1 strains: A/Indonesia/05/2005, A/Anhui/1/2005, and

A/Vietnam/1203/2004. The vaccine effectively generates an immune response that neutralizes the avian influenza virus in chickens and prevents productive replication in the host.

Safety issues of DNA vaccines

The major concerns with regard to safety of DNA vaccines are integration of the plasmid DNA into the host genome, adverse immunopathological effects, the formation of anti-DNA antibodies resulting in auto-immune disease and the use of novel molecular adjuvants. Moreover, for veterinary vaccines intended to be used in husbandry animals, food safety aspects also become an important issue. All new vaccine candidates should therefore be thoroughly tested in target animals, keeping in mind that for food producing animals, the products will be consumed. Finally, a further safety aspect of interest concerns the possible spread of genetic material to the environment, by the potential transformation of the environmental microflora with only a few copies of complete or fragmented plasmid. These are issues that need to be considered in the final scientific decisions underpinning the registration of vaccines. Major emphasis needs to be placed on aspects, such as the biodistribution of plasmid in vaccinated animals (Medjitna *et al.*, 2006).

a) Immediate post-vaccination reactions

After any vaccination a localized tissue reaction may be observed at the site of vaccine deposition. With DNA-vaccines, the administration of naked DNA without adjuvants gives very little tissue-reactions; even when the volume is large. If an adjuvant is included in the DNA-vaccine, the extent of tissue reactions will mainly depend on the tissue-damage created by the adjuvant (Parker *et al.*, 1999).

b) Systemic reactions

The level of systemic adverse reactions or toxicity seems to be very low after a DNA-vaccination with naked DNA in saline solution in any tissue. The adverse reactions produced by high endotoxin levels in a vaccine are well known from traditional vaccines and the precautions are similar for DNA-vaccines. Parker *et al.* (1999) found no systemic toxicity as evaluated by clinical pathology and histopathology and no adverse effects in terms of ophthalmology, body and organ weights, weight gain or food consumption that could be attributed to the vaccine.

c) Undesired immune response

When a consumer ingests the plasmids in meat from vaccinated animals, the question is raised whether an un-desired immune response is evoked in the consumer against the plasmid-encoded protein. In other words, is the consumer also"vaccinated" against the infective agent? Theoretically, the expression of plasmid DNA may be possible after oral intake, provided that the plasmid DNA "survives" through the gastric juice and reaches the intestines in a sufficiently large amount. Recently, different new approaches have been investigated in an attempt to overcome the gastric degradation and other barriers after oral administration of a DNA-vaccine, e.g. The PLG-encapsulation effectively protected the DNA against degradation and evoked IgA antibody responses (Jones *et al.,* 1997). Provided that there is no expression of irrelevant genes located on the plasmid, this topic is not relevant for the vaccinated animals.

d) Induction of anti-DNA antibody

The immunogenicity of DNA-vaccines is well established, but a concern has been raised regarding their potential to induce deleterious autoimmune responses, e.g. antibodies to mammalian DNA (Robertson *et al.,* 1994). The concerns are mainly based on the fact that the plasmid backbone of DNA-vaccines is of bacterial origin and thus has intrinsic immunostimulatory activity. Due to these immunomodulatory properties, bacterial DNA has the potential to stimulate normal mice to induce anti-mammalianDNA (anti-mDNA) auto-antibodies and as a result develop e.g. glomerulonephritis and renal dysfunction. There is no evidence to suspect that the inserted gene of a vaccine-plasmid in general should be more immunogenic than the rest of the plasmid. The level of auto-antibody production elicited by conventional DNA-vaccines is insufficient to induce active autoimmune disease in vaccinated animals (Mor *et al.,* 1997).

e) Induction of immunological tolerance

The specificity of the immune system is based on its ability to discriminate between self and non-self antigens. If the immune system does not possess the ability to react against a certain foreign antigen, the organism is tolerant and cannot mount an immune response against it. Experimental evidence suggests that recognition of foreign determinants is acquired at distinct ages of maturation, ranging from early gestation until days or weeks after birth (Mor, 2001). A bovine fetus, which is infected with Bovine Virus Diarrhea (BVD), is able to mount protective immunity and clear the infection in the last two thirds of the pregnancy. On the other hand, the calf will become immunologically tolerant and a persistent-infected carrier of the virus, if the fetus is infected during the first third of the pregnancy (Duffell *et al.*, 1985). There are qualitative and quantitative differences between the immune responses elicited by neonatal versus adult inoculation of DNA-vaccines. Although the magnitude of the immune response is generally smaller in neonates than in young and adult animals, a number of studies reported significant protection against infectious challenge carried out during adulthood.

f) Allergic reactions to antibiotic residues

During the production of plasmids in *E. coli*, an antibiotic resistance marker placed on the plasmid is used to select the bacteria that contain plasmids and kill the bacteria that do not posses a plasmid. The amount of antibiotic added to the bacterial solution at the beginning of fermentation is for instance 50 μg/ml of kanamycin or 100 μg/ml of ampicillin. The final product of the fermentation may therefore contain antibiotic residues, which if injected into an allergic recipient, may result in an anaphylactic reaction which may range from mild erythema or irritation to more severe systemic reactions and discomfort (Kutzler and Weiner, 2008).

g) Integration into chromosomal DNA

Integration of plasmid DNA into the recipient's genome appears the major point of attention of DNA vaccination. Integration may occur randomly or by homologous recombination. Integration could lead to activation of oncogenes, inactivation of tumor suppressor genes, or, when integrated into the chromosomal DNA of germ line cells, to vertical transmission (Kutzler and Weiner, 2008). However, there are no evidences of such consequence till date.

h) Germline and transplacental transmission

When plasmid is transmitted to the gonads, germ line chromosomal integration and germ line transmission could occur. Plasmid DNA may be detected in gonads shortly upon injection (Manam *et al.*, 2000) but integration of plasmid DNA into chromosomal germ line DNA has not been observed so far. These issues might need further investigation, especially if the DNA-vaccine is intended for pregnant animals.

i) Spread of genes to the environment

After a vaccination, only a small proportion of the injected plasmids is released from the injection site to systemic circulation and excreted to the intestinal contents (Zhang *et al.,* 2005). Bacteria in the intestines, the food and the environment can take up plasmids. The important genes in this respect are the antibiotic resistance genes present in most plasmids. However, antibiotic resistant bacteria are already naturally present in the environment. The uptake of plasmids happens with a very low frequency. The probability that a DNA-vaccination increases the risk of acquiring a disease caused by resistant bacteria seems negligible.

Application of Nucleic acid vaccines in viral diseases of veterinary importance

Veterinary vaccinology is a rapidly developing field. DNA vaccines have promoted a revolution in the concept of vaccination, which has been previously dominated by inactivated or live vaccines. Among many advantages, DNA vaccines also provide DIVA strategy, and hence vaccine-induced herd/flock immunity can be differentiated for effective sero-surveillance (Lee *et al.,* 2004). Table 3 presented the latest research development in the field of nucleic acid-based vaccination strategy for preventing various viral diseases of domestic animals as well as poultry in detail.

Table 3. DNA vaccines under trial for infectious viral diseases of veterinary importance

Host	Viral Diseases	Etiological agent	Protective antigen gene	References
Cattle	Bovine leukemia	Retrovirus	gp51; gp30	Brillowska *et al.* 1999
	Bovine rota virus	Rotavirus	VP4	Suradhat *et al.* 1997
	Infectious bovine rhinotracheitis	Bovine herpes virus	gC; gD	Gupta *et al.* 2001, Manoj *et al.* 2004
	Bovine viral diarrhea	Pestivirus	E2	Nobiron *et al.* 2003
	Foot and mouth disease	Picornavirus	VP1	Dong *et al.* 2005
Swine	Swine fever	Pestivirus	E2	Wienhold *et al.* 2005
	Pseudorabies	Herpes virus	gB; gC; gD	Gerdts *et al.* 1999, Dory *et al.* 2005
Canines	Parvoviral infections	Parvovirus	VP1; VP2	Jiang *et al.* 1998, Gupta *et al.* 2005
	Rabies	Rhabdovirus	gp gene	Rai *et al.* 2005 Gupta *et al.*, 2006
	Canine distemper	Morbilivirus	HA; F	Sixt *et al.* 1998
Equines	Equine influenza	Influenza virus	HA	Lunn *et al.* 1999
	Equine herpes infection	Herpes virus	gB; gC; gD	Minke *et al.* 2006
Poultry	Avian influenza	Influenza virus	HA	Kodihalli *et al.* 2000
	Newcastle disease	Avian paramyxovirus	HN; F	Loke *et al.* 2005
	Infectious bronchitis	Coronavirus	N; S1	Seo *et al.* 1997
	Infectious bursal disease	Avibirnavirus	VP2	Li *et al.* 2006
	Chicken infectious anemia	Gyrovirus	VP1 and VP2	Senthil Kumar *et al.* 2004

Licensed DNA plasmid products for animal health

Currently three DNA vaccines have been licensed for veterinary use :

a) West Nile- Innovator DNA

Wyeth Fort Dodge Laboratories (Fort Dodge, IA), in conjunction with the Centers for Disease Control and Prevention (Atlanta, GA), developed a DNA vaccine to protect horses from West Nile virus and this became the first DNA vaccine licensed by the USDA (Holl and Redding, 2005) in 2005 but is not commercially available. The vaccine contains recombinant plasmid (pCBWN), which expresses the WN virus prM (pre-membrane) and E (envelope) structural proteins. Vaccinated horses showed development of neutralising antibodies and protection against challenge (Davis *et al.*, 2001). The presence of maternally-derived antibodies does not prevent induction of specific immunity in the foals (Chiang *et al.*, 2005). Two doses of 2 ml vaccine are usually used for intramuscular vaccination of healthy horses 8 months of age or older as an aid in the prevention of viremia caused by West Nile virus. A second 2 ml dose is given 2 to 4 weeks after the first dose. The animal is then re-vaccinated annually with a 2 ml dose.

b) Canine Melanoma Vaccine Oncept™

The Merial Memorial Sloan-Kettering Cancer Center (New York, NY) and the Animal Medical Center (New York, NY) developed a DNA vaccine that is conditional licensed in 2007 to treat and prevent canine melanoma (Bergman, 2007, Merial, 2007). This therapeutic vaccine uses DNA expressing the human tyrosinase gene. The tyrosinase encoded by the xenogeneic (different-species) DNA used in this vaccine is homologous to canine tyrosinase and has been shown to stimulate an immune response to canine melanoma cells expressing tyrosinase. The ability to prolong the lives of dogs with even advanced disease provides a degree of effectiveness for immunotherapy greater than that seen with other immunotherapeutic vaccines in development. The therapeutic vaccine is administered transdermally in four doses biweekly. Each 0.4 mL dose is injected in the medial thigh using the Canine transdermal device (VET JET).

c) Infectious haematopoietic necrosis virus (Apex-IHN™)

Apex®-IHN is a Purified pUK-ihnG nucleic acid vaccine for use by salmon farms in the prevention of infectious hematopoietic necrosis virus (IHNV) disease (Lorenzen and LaPatra, 2005, Vical Inc., 2005). It was developed by Novartis based on technology licensed from Vical. Apex®-IHN received licensure from the Canadian Food Inspection Agency (CFIA) in 2005, the first commercial DNA vaccine to achieve approval for sale and use in Canada, where it is currently marketed by Novartis Aqua Health. It recommends injecting the vaccine at a dose of 1ìg/fish, delivered in a volume of 0.05mL saline one-time intramuscularly in the area immediately anterior and lateral to the dorsal fin (epaxial muscle) to young fish at the hatchery. It is effective in generating a robust immune response to prevent such outbreaks.

Conclusions and Future Prospects

Vaccination with DNA is one of the most promising novel immunization techniques against pathogens, for which conventional vaccination regimens have been less effective. DNA vaccines, nick named 'immunological silver bullet', have now become well established in clinical trials after about 20 years of experimentation. In small experimental animals, the milder host impedance has permitted the DNA vaccines to induce lasting protective effects in contrast to much tougher host barriers in large animals. Significant efforts have been put forward to identify methods of enhancing the immune response of plasmid DNA in higher mammals, with the use of immune modulators, cytokines and co-stimulatory molecules. If the potency is improved, plasmid DNA vaccines, having numerous advantages, can be useful for the active immunization against infectious diseases of animals. Efforts should be targeted towards improving their delivery or to increase their immunogenic potential. Poor cellular uptake and rapid in vivo degradation of plasmid DNA has to be taken into account and novel delivery systems has to be developed along with the optimization of the plasmid vector. The major challenge in future is the improvement of the transfection efficiency of the DNA vaccines. Gene gun and electroporation can increase transfection and improve immune responses significantly, but these technologies have not yet advanced to routine use in animals. Another promising approach is the development of microparticles as delivery systems or the non-invasive plasmid DNA immunization. The cost of the vaccine is another important issue. Plasmid purification is still expensive and the amounts injected needs to be reduced, if DNA vaccination is to be considered in breeding systems.

In nutshell, it can be concluded that the current scenario is much promise regarding the development of effective, safe and economically viable nucleic acid vaccines.

References

Akira, S., S. Uematsu and O. Takeuchi (2006). Pathogen recognition and innate immunity. *Cell*, **124**: 783-801.

Andrew, M.E., C.J. Morrissy, C. Lenghaus, P.G. Oke, K.W. Sproat, A.L.M. Hodgson, M.A. Johnson and B.E.H. Coupar (2000). Protection of pigs against classical swine fever with DNA-delivered gp55. *Vaccine*, **18**: 1932-1938.

Babiuk, S., M.E. Baca-Estrada, M. Foldvari, D.M. Middleton, D. Rabussay, G. Widera and L.A. Babiuk (2004). Increased gene expression and inflammatory cell infiltration caused by electroporation are both important for improving the efficacy of DNA vaccines. *J. Biotechnol.*, **110**: 1-10.

Babiuk, S., M.E. Baca-Estrada, M. Foldvari, L. Baizer, R. Stout, M. Storms, D. Rabussay, G. Widera and L. Babiuk (2003) Needle-free topical electroporation improves gene expression from plasmids administered in porcine skin. *Mol. Ther.*, **8**: 992–998.

Babiuk, S., S. van Drunen Littel-van den Hurk and L.A. Babiuk (2006). Delivery of DNA Vaccines Using Electroporation *In*: Saltzman, W.M., H. Shen and J.L. Brandsma (eds.) DNA Vaccines: Methods and Protocols, 2nd ed., Humana Press, New Jersay, USA, pp. 73-74.

Barry, M.E., D. Pinto-Gonzalez, F.M. Orson, G.J. McKenzie, G.R. Petry and M.A. Barry (1999). Role of endogenous endonucleases and tissue site in transfection and CpG-mediated immune activation after naked DNA injection. *Hum. Gene. Ther.*, **10**: 2461-80.

Beard, C., Ward, G., Rieder, E., Chinsangaram, J., Grubman, M.J. and Mason, P.W. (1999) Development of DNA vaccines for foot-and-mouth disease, evaluation of vaccines encoding replicating and non-replicating nucleic acids in swine. J. Biotechnol. **73**: 243-249.

Bergman, P. J. (2007). Anti-cancer vaccines. *Vet. Clin. North Am. Small Anim. Pract.*, **37**: 1111-1119.

Boretti, F.S., C.M. Leutenegger, C. Mislin, R. Hofmannlehmann, S. Konig, M. Schroff, C. Junghans, D. Fehr, S.W. Huettner, A. Habel, J.N. Flynn, A. Aubert, N.C. Pedersen, B. Wittig and H. Lutz (2000). Protection against FIV challenge infection by genetic vaccination using minimalistic DNA constructs for FIV env gene and feline IL-12 expression. *AIDS*, **14**: 1749-1757.

Brillowska, A., S. Dabrowski, J. Rulka, P. Kubis, E. Buzala and J. Kur (1999). Protection of cattle against bovine leukemia virus (BLV) infection could be attained by DNA vaccination. *Acta Biochemistry Poland*, **46**: 971-976.

Cardon, L. R., C. Burge, D.A. Clayton and S. Karlin (1994). Pervasive CpG suppression in animal mitochondrial genomes. *Proc. Natl. Acad. Sci. U. S A.,* **91**: 3799–3803.

Cherpillod, P., A. Tipold, M. Griotwenk, C. Cardozo, I. Schmid, R. Fatzer, M. Schobesberger, R. Zurbriggen, L. Bruckner, F. Roch, M. Vandevelde, R. Wittek and A. Zurbriggen (2000). DNA vaccine encoding nucleocapsid and surface proteins of wild type canine distemper virus protects its natural host against distemper. *Vaccine,* **18**: 2927-2936.

Chiang, Y.W., C.M. Jennen, T.M. Holt, C.P. Waldbillig, D.K. Hathaway, N.J. Jennings, T. Ng and H.J. Chu (2005). Demonstration of efficacy of a West Nile virus DNA vaccine in foals. 51st Annual Convention of the American Association of Equine Practitioners, Seattle, Washington, USA, **51**, IVIS Document No. P2627.1205.

Christensen, D., K. S. Korsholm, I. Rosenkrands, T. Lindenstrom, P. Andersen, and E. M. Agger (2007).Cationic liposomes as vaccine adjuvants. *Expert Rev. Vaccines,* **6**: 785-796.

Cui, Z. and R.J. Mumper (2003). Microparticles and nanoparticles as delivery systems for DNA vaccines. *Crit. Rev. Ther. Drug Carrier Syst.,* **20**: 103-37.

Davis, N.L., I.J. Caley, K.W. Brown, M.R. Betts, D.M. Irlbeck, K.M. McGrath, M.J. Connell, D.C. Montefiori, J.A. Frelinger, R. Swanstrom, P.R. Johnson and R.E. Johnston (2001).West Nile virus recombinant DNA vaccine protects mouse and horse from virus challenge and expresses *in vitro* a non-infectious recombinant antigen that can be used in enzyme-linked immunosorbent assays. *J. Virol.,* **75**: 4040–4047.

De Smedt, S.C., J. Demeester and W.E. Hennink (2000). Cationic polymer based gene delivery systems. *Pharm. Res.,* **17**: 113-126.

Dhama, K., M. Mahendran, P.K. Gupta and A. Rai (2008). DNA vaccines and their applications in veterinary practice: current perspectives. *Vet. Res. Commun.,* **32**: 341-356.

Dong, J.J., Y.L. Wang, Y.G. Zhang, X.P. Fu, L. Pan, Y.Z. Fang, S.T. Jiang, B.Q. Wang and W.X. Wang (2005). Construction of recombinant plasmid with VP1 genes against Asia I FMDV and elementary analysis of its immunological activity. *Chinese J. Vet. Sci. Technolo.,* **35:** 461–464.

Doria-Rose, N.A. and N.L. Haigwood (2003). DNA vaccine strategies: candidates for immune modulation and immunization regimens. *Methods,* **31**: 207-216.

Dory, D., V. Beven, A.M. Torche, S. Bougeard, R. Cariolet and A. Jestin (2005). CpG motif in ATCGAT hexamer improves DNA-vaccine efficiency against lethal Pseudorabies virus infection in pigs. *Vaccine,* **23**: 4532–4540.

Duffell, S. J. and J. W. Harkness (1985). Bovine virus diarrhoea-mucosal disease infection in cattle. *Vet. Rec.*, **117**: 240-245.

Dufour, V. (2001). DNA vaccines: new applications for veterinary medicine. *Vet. Sci. Tomorrow*, **2**: 1-25.

Dufour, V., S. Chevallier, R. Cariolet, S. Somasundaram, F. Lefèvre, A. Jestin and E. Albina (2000). Induction of porcine cytokine mRNA expression after DNA immunization and pseudorabies virus infection. *J. Interferon Cytokine Res.*, **20**: 885-890.

Dunham, S.P. (2002). The application of nucleic acid vaccines in veterinary medicine. *Res. Vet. Sci.*, **73**: 9–16.

Dupuis, M., K. Denis-Mize, C. Woo, C. Goldbeck, M.J. Selby, M. Chen, G.R. Otten, J.B. Ulmer, J.J. Donnelly, G. Ott and D.M. McDonald (2000). Distribution of DNA vaccines determines their immunogenicity after intramuscular injection in mice. *J. Immunol.*, **165**: 2850-2858.

Felgner, P.L., T.R. Gadek, M. Holm, R. Roman, H.W. Chan, M. Wenz, J.P. Northrop, G.M. Ringold and M. Danielsen (1987). Lipofection: a highly efficient, lipidmediated DNA-transfection procedure. *Proc. Natl. Acad. Sci. U. S. A.*, **84**: 7413–7417.

Fodor, I., E. Horvath, N. Fodor, E. Nagy, A. Rencendorsh, V.N. Vakharia and S.K. Dube (1999). Induction of protective immunity in chickens immunised with plasmid DNA encoding bursal disease virus antigens. *Acta Vet. Hung.*, **47**: 481-492.

Fuller, D.H., M.M. Corb, S. Barnett, K. Steamer and J.R. Haynes (1997). Enhancement of immunodeficiency virus specific immune responses in DNA immunized rhesus macaques. *Vaccine*, **15**: 924-926.

Funhoff, A.M., C.F. van Nostrum, A.P.C.A. Janssen, M.H.A.M. Fens, D.J.A. Crommelin and W.E. Hennink (2004). Polymer side-chain degradation as a tool to control the destabilization of polyplexes. *Pharm. Res.*, **21**: 170-176.

Fynan, E.F., R.G. Webster, D.H. Fuller, J.R. Haynes, J.C. Santoro and J.L. Robinson (1993). DNA: Vaccines: Protective immunizations by parental, mucosal and gene-gun inoculations. *Proc. Natl. Acad. Sci. USA*, **90**: 11478-11482.

Gaumet, M., R. Gurny and F. Delie (2009). Localization and quantification of biodegradable particles in an intestinal cell model: the influence of particle size. *Eur. J. Pharm. Sci.*, **36**: 465-473.

Gerdts, V., A. Jons and T.C. Mettenleiter (1999). Potency of an experimental DNA vaccine against Aujeszky's disease in pigs. *Vet. Microbiol.*, **66**: 1–13.

Goh, S.L., N. Murthy, M. Xu and J.M.J. Frechet (2004). Cross-linked microparticles as carriers for the delivery of plasmid DNA for vaccine development. *Bioconjug. Chem.*, **15**: 467-474.

Griot, C., C. Moser, P. Cherpillod, L. Bruckner, R. Wittek, A. Zurbriggen and R. Zurbriggen (2003). Early DNA vaccination of puppies against canine distemper in the presence of maternally derived immunity. *Vaccine*, **22**: 651-655.

Gupta, P.K., A. Rai, N. Rai, A. Raut and S. Chauhan (2005). Cloning of canine parvovirus VP2 gene and its use as DNA vaccine in dogs. *Current Sci.*, **88**: 778–782

Gupta, P.K., M. Saini, L.K. Gupta, V.D. Rao, S.K. Bandyopadhyay, G. Butchaiah, G.K. Garg and S.K. Garg (2001). Induction of immune responses in cattle with a DNA vaccine encoding glycoprotein C of bovine herpesvirus-1. *Vet. Microbiol.*, **78**: 293-305.

Gupta, P.K., S. Sharma, S.S. Walunj, A.A. Patil, A. Rai and M. Saini (2006). A DNA vaccine that encodes rabies virus glycoprotein lacking transmembrane domain enhances antibody response but not protection. *Acta Virologica*, **50**: 87–92.

Gurunathan, S., D.M. Klinman and R.A. Seder (2000). DNA vaccines: immunology, application, and optimization. *Annual Rev. Immunol.*, **18**: 927–974.

Hagstrom, J.E., J. Hegge, G. Zhang, M. Noble, V. Budker, D.L. Lewis, H. Herweijer and J.A. Wolff (2004). A facile nonviral method for delivering genes and siRNAs to skeletal muscle of mammalian limbs. *Mol Ther.*, **10**: 386–398.

Harpin, S., D.J. Hurley, M. Mbikay, B. Talbot and Y. Elazhary (1999) Vaccination of cattle with a DNA plasmid encoding the bovine viral diarrhoea virus major glycoprotein E2. *J. Gen. Virol.*, **80**: 3137-3144.

Hartmann, G., R.D. Weeratna, Z.K. Ballas, P. Payette, S. Blackwell, I. Suparto, W.L. Rasmussen, M. Waldschmidt, D. Sajuthi, R.H. Purcell, H.L. Davis and A.M. Krieg (2000). Delineation of a CpG phosphorothioate oligodeoxynucleotide for activating primate immune responses in vitro and in vivo. *J. Immunol.*, **164**: 1617–1624.

Hedley, M.L., J. Curley and R. Urban (1998). Microspheres containing plasmid-encoded antigens elicit cytotoxic T-cell responses. *Nat. Med.*, **4**: 365-368.

Holl, S., and J. Redding (2005). USDA issues license for West Nile virus DNA vaccine for horses. http://www.aphis.usda.gov/lpa/news/2005/07/wnvdna_vs.html Accessed July 2008.

Hosie, M.J. and O. Jarret (1999). Analysis of the protective immunity induced by feline immunodeficiency virus vaccination. *Adv. Vet. Med.*, **41**: 325-332.

Ioannou, X. P., S.M. Gomis, B. Karvonen, R. Hecker, L.A. Babiuk, and S. van Drunen Littel-van den Hurk (2002). CpG-containing oligodeoxynucleotides, in combination with conventional adjuvants, enhance the magnitude and change the bias of the immune responses to a herpesvirus glycoprotein. *Vaccine*, **21**: 127–137.

Ito, Y. (1960). A tumor reducing factor extracted by phenol from papillomatous tissue of cotton tail rabbits. *Virology*, 12: 596-601.

Jadav, S.K., K.S. Reddy, B.R. Rashmi, H.J. Dechamma, K. Ganesh, V.V.S. Suryanarayana and G.R. Reddy (2011). A secretary DNA vaccine construct delivered by PLG micro particles against foot and mouth disease in guinea pigs. *Res. Vet. Sci.*, **91**: 86-89.

Jiang, W., H.J. Baker, L.J. Swango, J. Schorr, M.J. Self and B.F. Smith (1998). Nucleic acid immunization protects dogs against challenge with virulent canine parvovirus. *Vaccine*, **16**: 601-607.

Jilek, S., H.P. Merkle and E. Walter (2005). DNA-loaded biodegradable microparticles as vaccine delivery systems and their interaction with dendritic cells. *Adv. Drug Deliv. Rev.*, **57**: 377-390.

Jones, D. H., S. Corris, S. McDonald, J. C. Clegg, and G. H. Farrar (1997). Poly (DL-lactide-co-glycolide)-encapsulated plasmid DNA elicits systemic and mucosal antibody responses to encoded protein after oral administration. *Vaccine*, **15**: 814-817.

Kodihalli, S., D.L. Kobasa and R.G. Webster (2000). Strategies for inducing protection against avian A virus subtypes with DNA vaccines. *Vaccine*, **18**: 2592–2599.

Krieg, A. M., A.K. Yi, J. Schorr and H.L. Davis (1998). The role of CpG dinucleotides in DNA vaccines. *Trends Microbiol.*, **6**: 23–27.

Kutzler, M.A. and D.B. Weiner (2008). DNA vaccines: ready for prime time?. *Nature Rev. Genetics*, **9**: 776-788.

Landolt, G.A., S.B. Hussey, K. Kreutzer, A. Quintana and D.P. Lunn (2010). Low-dose DNA vaccination into the submandibular lymph nodes in ponies. *Vet. Rec.*, **167**: 302-303.

Lappalainen, K, I. Jaaskelainen, K. Syrjanen, A. Urtti and S. Syrjanen (1994). Comparison of cell proliferation and toxicity assays using two cationic liposomes. *Pharm. Res.*, **11**: 1127-1131.

Lee, C.W., D.A. Senne and D.L. Suarez, D.L. (2004). Generation of re-assortant influenza vaccines by reverse genetics that allows utilization of a DIVA (Differentiating Infected from Vaccinated Animals) strategy for the control of avian influenza. *Vaccine*, **22**: 3175–3181.

Lehmann, M.J. and G. Sczakiel (2005). Spontaneous uptake of biologically active recombinant DNA by mammalian cells via a selected DNA segment. *Gene Ther.*, **12**: 446-451.

Li, L., W.H. Fang, J.R. Li, L. Fang, Y.W. Huang and L. Yu (2006). Oral DNA vaccination with polyprotein gene of IBDV delivered by attenuated

Salmonella elicits protective immune response in chickens. *Vaccine*, **24**: 5919–5927.

Liang, R., J.V. van den Hurk, L.A. Babiuk and S. van Drunen Littel-van den Hurk (2006). Priming with DNA encoding E2 and boosting with E2 protein formulated with CpG oligodeoxy-nucleotides induces strong immune responses and protection from Bovine viral diarrhea virus in cattle. *J. Gen. Virol.*, **87**: 2971–2982.

Liu, F., Y. Song and D. Liu (1999). Hydrodynamics-based transfection in animals by systemic administration of plasmid DNA. *Gene Ther.*, **6**: 1258–1266.

Liu, Li-Juan, S. Watabe, J. Yang, K. Hamajima, N. Ishii, E. Hagiwara, K. Onari, K.Q. Xin and K. Okuda (2001). Topical application of HIV DNA vaccine with cytokine-expression plasmids induces strong antigen-specific immune responses. *Vaccine*, **20**: 42-48.

Liu, M.A. (2003). DNA vaccines: a review. *J. Internal Med.*, **253**: 402–410.

Loehr, B.I., P. Willson, L.A. Babiuk and S. van Drunen Littel-van Den Hurk (2000). Gene gunmediated DNA immunization primes development of mucosal immunity against bovine herpesvirus 1 in cattle. *J. Virol.*, **74**: 6077-6086.

Loehr, B.I., R. Rankin, R. Pontarollo, T. King, P. Willson, L.A. Babiuk and S. van Drunen Littel-van den Hurk (2001). Suppository-mediated DNA immunization induces mucosal immunity against bovine herpesvirus-1 in cattle. *Virology*, **289**: 327–333.

Loke, C.F., A.R. Omar, A.R. Raha and K. Yusoff (2005). Improved protection from velogenic Newcastle disease virus challenge following multiple immunizations with plasmid DNA encoding for F and HN genes. *Vet. Immunol. Immunopathol.*, **106**: 259–267.

Lorenzen, N., and S. E. LaPatra (2005). DNA vaccines for aquacultured fish. *Rev. Sci. Tech.* **24**: 201–213.

Luby-Phelps, K. (2000). Cytoarchitecture and physical properties of cytoplasm: volume, viscosity, diffusion, intracellular surface area. *Int. Rev. Cytol.*, **192**: 189-221.

Ludtke, J.J., M.G. Sebestyen and J.A. Wolff (2002). The effect of cell division on the cellular dynamics of microinjected DNA and dextran. *Mol. Ther.*, **5**: 579-588.

Lunn, D.P., G. Soboll, B.R. Schram, J. Quass, M.W. McGregor, R.J. Drape, M.D. Macklin, D.E. McCabe, W.F. Swain and C.W. Olsen (1999). Antibody responses to DNA vaccination of horses using the influenza virus hemagglutinin gene. *Vaccine*, **17**: 2245–2258.

Macklin, M.D., D. McCabe, M.W. McGregor, V. Neumann, T. Meyer, R. Callan, V.S. Hinshaw and W.F. Swain (1998). Immunization of pigs with a particle-mediated DNA vaccine to influenza A virus protects against challenge with homologous virus. *J. Virol.*, **72**: 1491-1496.

Manam, S., B.J. Ledwith, A.B. Barnum, P.J. Troilo, C.J. Pauley, L.B. Harper, T.G. Griffiths, Z. Niu, L. Denisova, T.T. Follmer, S.J. Pacchione, Z. Wang, C.M. Beare, W.J. Bagdon and W.W. Nichols (2000). Plasmid DNA vaccines: tissue distribution and effects of DNA sequence, adjuvants and delivery method on integration into host DNA. *Intervirology*, **43**: 273-281.

Manoj, S., P.J. Griebel, L.A. Babiuk and S. van Drunen Littel-van den Hurk (2004). Modulation of immune responses to bovine herpesvirus-1 in cattle by immunization with a DNA vaccine encoding glycoprotein D as a fusion protein with bovine CD154. *Immunology*, **112**: 328–338.

Martínez-Gómez, J.M., P. Johansen, I. Erdmann, G. Senti, R. Crameri and T.M. Kündig (2009). Intralymphatic injections as a new administration route for allergen-specific immunotherapy. *Int. Arch. Allergy Immunol.*, **150**: 59-65.

Medjitna, T.D., C. Stadler, L. Bruckner, C. Griot and H.P. Ottiger (2006). DNA vaccines: safety aspect assessment and regulation. *Dev. Biol.*, **126**: 261-270.

Meeusen, E.N.T., J. Walker, A. Peters, P.P. Pastoret and G. Jungersen (2007). Current Status of Veterinary Vaccines. *Clin. Microbiol. Rev.*, **20**: 489–510.

Merial (2007). Merial's new vaccine treats deadly cancer in dogs. http://us.merial.com/merial_corporate/news/press_releases/03-26-2007_melanoma_consumer.asp

Minke, J.M., L. Fischer, P. Baudu, P.M. Guigal, T. Sindle, J.A. Mumford and J.C. Audonnet (2006). Use of DNA and recombinant canarypox viral vectors for equine herpes virus vaccination. *Vet. Immunol. Immunopathol.*, **111**: 47–57.

Monteil, M., M.F. Le Potier, J. Guillotin, R. Cariolet, C. Houdayer and M. Eloit (1996) Genetic immunization of seronegative one-day-old piglets against pseudorabies induces neutralizing antibodies but not protection and is ineffective in piglets from immune dams. *Vet. Res.*, **27**: 443-452.

Mor, G. and M. Eliza (2001). Plasmid DNA vaccines. Immunology, tolerance, and autoimmunity. *Mol. Biotechnol.*, **19**: 245-250.

Mor, G., M. Singla, A. D. Steinberg, S. L. Hoffman, K. Okuda, and D. M. Klinman (1997). Do DNA vaccines induce autoimmune disease? *Hum. Gene Ther.*, **8**: 293-300.

Newman, K.D., P. Elamanchili, G.S. Kwon and J. Samuel (2002). Uptake of poly(D,L-lactic-co-glycolic acid) microspheres by antigen-presenting cells in vivo. *J. Biomed. Mater. Res.*, **60**: 480-486.

Nguyen, D.N., J.G. Jordan, M.C. Juliana, L. Robert and G.A. Daniel (2008). Polymeric Materials for Gene Delivery and DNA Vaccination. *Adv. Mater.*, **20**: 1–21.

Nobiron, I., I. Thompson, J. Brownlie and M.E. Collins (2003). DNA vaccination against bovine viral diarrhoea virus induces humoral and cellular responses in cattle with evidence for protection against viral challenge. *Vaccine*, **21**: 2082–2092.

Oshop, G.L., S. Elankumaran and R.A. Heckert (2002). DNA vaccination in avian. *Vet. Immunol. Immunopathol.*, **89**: 1–12.

Osorio, J.E., C.C. Tomlinson, R.S. Frank, E.J. Haanes, K. Rushlow, J.R. Haynes and D.T. Stinchcomb (1999). Immunization of dogs and cats with a DNA vaccine against rabies virus. *Vaccine*, **17**: 1109-1116.

Oster, C.G., N. Kim, L. Grode, L. Barbu-Tudoran, A.K. Schaper, S.H.E. Kaufmann and T. Kissel (2005). Cationic microparticles consisting of poly (lactide-co-glycolide) and polyethylenimine as carriers systems for parental DNA vaccination. *J.Control Release*, **104:** 359-377.

Parker, S. E., F. Borellini, M. L. Wenk, P. Hobart, S. L. Hoffman, R. Hedstrom, T. Le, and J. A. Norman (1999). Plasmid DNA malaria vaccine: tissue distribution and safety studies in mice and rabbits. *Hum.Gene Ther.*, **10**: 741-758.

Pavlin, D., N. Tozon, G. Sersa, A. Pogacnik and M. Cemazar (2008). Efficient Electrotransfection into Canine Muscle. Technology in Cancer Research and Treatment, 7(1), www.tcrt.org, (Open Access Article).

Pertmer, T.M., T.R. Roberts and J.R. Haynes (1996). Influenza virus nucleoprotein-specific immunoglobulin G subclass and cytokine responses elicited by DNA vaccination are dependent on the route of vector DNA delivery. *J. Virol.*, **70**: 6119-6125.

Petrini, S., G. Ramadori, A. Corradi, P. Borghetti, G. Lombardi, R. Villa, E. Bottarelli, A. Guercio, A. Amici and M. Ferrari (2011). Evaluation of safety and efficacy of DNA vaccines against bovine herpesvirus-1 (BoHV-1) in calves. Comp. Immunol. Microbiol. Infect. Dis., **34**: 3-10.

Rai, N., P. Kaushik and A. Rai (2005). Development of rabies DNA vaccine using a recombinant plasmid. *Acta Virologica*, **49**: 207–210.

Rao, S. S., D. Styles, W. Kong, C. Andrews, J. P. Gorres and G. J. Nabel (2009). A gene-based avian influenza vaccine in poultry. *Poult. Sci.*, **88**: 860-866.

Rawat, M., D. Singh, S. Saraf and S. Saraf (2007). An overview of biochemical aspects of DNA vaccines. *Asian J. Biochem.*, **2**: 208-223.

Reyes-Sandoval, A. and H.C. Ertl (2001).DNA vaccines. *Curr Mol Med.*, **1**: 217-243.

Robertson, J. S. (1994). Safety considerations for nucleic acid vaccines. *Vaccine,* **12**: 1526-1528.

Roques, C., E. Fattal and Y. Fromes (2009). Comparison of toxicity and transfection efficiency of amphiphilic block copolymers and polycationic polymers in striated muscles. *J. Gene Med.,* **11**: 240-249.

Ross, D.W. (2002). *Introduction to Molecular Medicine.* 3rd edition, Springer-Verlag, New York, USA, pp. 66-67.

Satkauskas, S., F. Andre, M.F. Bureau, D. Scherman, D. Miklavcic and L.M. Mir (2005). Electrophoretic Component of Electric Pulses Determines the Efficacy of In Vivo DNA Electrotransfer. *Hum. Gene Ther.,* **10**: 1194-1201.

Schrijver, R.S., J.P. Langedijk, G.M. Keil, W.G. Middel, M. Maris-Veldhuis, J.T. Van Oirschot and F.A. Rijsewijk (1998) Comparison of DNA application methods to reduce BRSV shedding in cattle. *Vaccine,* **16:** 130-134.

Senthil Kumar, N., J.M. Kataria, K. Dhama, N. Bhardwaj, S.A. Sylvester and S. Rahul (2004). Development of DNA vaccine against chicken anemia virus simultaneously using its VP1 and VP2 proteins. Paper Presented in XII Conference of IPSA and National Symposium, April 7-9, 2004 at Himachal Pradesh Krishi Vishwavidyalya, Palampur. pp. 152.

Senti, G., P. Johansen and T.M. Kündig (2009). Intralymphatic immunotherapy. *Curr. Opin. Allergy Clin. Immunol.,* **9**: 537-543.

Seo, S.H., L. Wang, R. Smith and E.W. Collisson (1997). The carboxyl-terminal 120-residue polypeptide of IB virus nucleocapsid induces CTLs and protects chickens from acute infection. *J. Virol.,* **71**: 7889–7894.

Sin, J.I., M. Bagarazzi, C. Pachuk and D.B. Weiner (1999). DNA priming-protein boosting enhances both antigen-specific antibody and Th1-type cellular immune responses in a murine herpes simplex virus-2 gD vaccine model. *DNA and Cell Biol.,* **18**: 771-779.

Sixt, N., A. Cardoso, A. Vallier, J. Fayolle, R. Buckland and T.F. Wild (1998). CD virus DNA vaccination induces humoral and cellular immunity and protects against a lethal intracerebral challenge. *J. Virol.,* **72**: 8472–8476.

Somasundaram, C., H. Takamatsu, C. Andréoni, J.C. Audonnet, L. Fisher, F. Lefèvre and B. Charley (1999). Enhanced protective response and immuno-adjuvant effects of porcine GM-CSF on DNA vaccination of pigs against Aujeszky's disease virus. *Vet. Immunol. Immunopathol.* **70**: 277-287.

Suradhat, S., D. Yoo, L.A. Babiuk, P. Griebel and M.E. Baca-Estrada (1997). DNA immunization with a bovine rotavirus VP4 gene induces a Th1-like immune response in mice. *Viral Immunol.,* **10**: 117–127.

van Drunen Littel-van den Hurk, S., M. Snider, P. Thompson, L. Latimer and L.A. Babiuk (2008). Strategies for induction of protective immunity to bovine herpesvirus-1 in newborn calves with maternal antibodies. *Vaccine,* **26**: 3103-3111.

van Drunen Littel-van den Hurk, S., R.P. Braun, P.J. Lewis, B.C. Karvonen, L.A. Babiuk and P.J. Griebel (1999) Immunization of neonates with DNA encoding a bovine herpesvirus glycoprotein is effective in the presence of maternal antibodies. *Viral Immunol.,* **12**: 67-77.

van Rooij, E.M., B.L. Haagmans, Y.E. de Visser, M.G. de Bruin, W. Boersma and A.T. Bianchi (1998). Effect of vaccination route and composition of DNA vaccine on the induction of protective immunity against pseudorabies infection in pigs. *Vet. Immunol. Immunopathol.,* **66**: 113-126.

Vaughan, E.E. and D.A. Dean (2006). Intracellular trafficking of plasmids during transfection is mediated by microtubules. *Mol. Ther.,* **13**: 422-428.

Vical Inc. (2005). Vical announces marketing approval of DNA vaccine for salmon. Goliath, The Gale Group, Cengage Learning, Farmington Hills, MI. http://goliath.ecnext.com/coms2/summary_0199-4481412_ITM Accessed August 2008.

Vives, E., J. Schmidt and A. Pelegrin (2008). Cell-penetrating and cell-targeting peptides in drug delivery. *Biochim. Biophys. Acta,* **1786**: 126-138.

Wienhold, D., E. Armengol, A. Marquardt, C. Marquardt, H. Voigt, M. Buttner, A. Saalmuller and E. Pfaff (2005). Immuno-modulatory effect of plasmids co-expressing cytokines in classical swine fever virus subunit gp55/E2-DNA vaccination. *Vet. Res.,* **36**: 571–587.

Winegar, R.A., J.A. Monforte, K.D. Suing, O.L. Kg, C.J. Rudd and J.T. Macgregor (1996). Determination of tissue distribution of an intramuscular plasmid vaccine using PCR and in situ DNA hybridization. *Hum. Gene Ther.,* **7**: 2185-2194.

Wolff, J.A., R.W. Malone, P. Williams, W. Chong, G. Acsadi, A. Jani and P.L. Felgner (1990). Direct gene transfer into mouse muscle *in vivo. Science,* **247**: 1465–1468.

Wolfgang W.L., Y. Han and P.R. Nicholas (1999). DNA and RNA-based vaccines: principles, progress and prospects. *Vaccine,* **18**: 765–777.

Zhang, H.Y., S.H. Sun, Y.J. Guo, Z.H. Chen, L. Huang, Y.J. Gao, B. Wan, W.J. Zhu, G.X. Xu and J.J. Wang (2005). Tissue distribution of a plasmid DNA containing epitopes of foot-and-mouth disease virus in mice. *Vaccine,* **23**: 5632-40.

□□□

Chapter 7

Ovarian Apoptosis-Boon and the Bane

JAFRIN ARA AHMED[1] AND NAWAB NASHIRUDDULLAH[2]

[1] Division of Veterinary Physiology & Biochemistry
[2] Division of Veterinary Pathology
Faculty of Veterinary Sciences & Animal Husbandry,
Sher-e-Kashmir University of Agricultural University Sciences & Technology-Jammu, RS Pura-181102, Jammu & Kashmir, India

Introduction

Isaac Asimov once noted: *"Life is pleasant. Death is peaceful. It's the transition that's troublesome"*

The term 'apoptosis' was coined by Kerr *et al.* (1972) to describe the process of programmed cell death in multicellular organisms. Functionally, apoptosis is thought to play a major role in tissue morphogenesis during development, in the physiological regulation of cell number, and in mediating the cellular response to adversity. To induce cell-death, apoptotic signals must cause regulatory proteins to initiate the apoptosis pathway. Several proteins are involved, but two main methods of regulation have been identified: (i) directly transduce the extrinsic signals via adaptor proteins to the apoptotic mechanisms, or (ii) intrinsic signals targeting the mitochondrial functionality. The extrinsic pathway (death receptor-mediated apoptotic events) is activated by tumour necrosis factor family receptors triggered by pro-apoptotic ligands (such as Apo2L/TRAIL and CD95L/FASL) binding to their cognate receptors (DR4/DR5and CD95/FAS, respectively). This induces the clustering of these receptors followed by recruitment of FAS associated death domain (FADD) and caspase 8 or 10, which constitute the death-inducing signalling complex. In contrast, the intrinsic apoptotic process (mitochondria-mediated apoptotic events) represents a default pathway for cells that are suffering from disruption of cellular homeostasis as a consequence of stress induced by a wide variety of factors including attack by reactive oxygen species (ROS), detachment from extracellular matrix, heat, hypoxia,

γ-irradiation, DNAdamage, or just lack of pro-survival factors (Aitken *et al.*, 2011). Alternatively, an increase in calcium concentration within a cell by toxins also initiates apoptosis *via* calcium binding protease calpain.

Apoptotic Proteins

Apoptosis is regulated by the interplay of the pro - and anti-apoptotic (pro-survival) factors, involving chiefly members of the B-cell lymphoma/leukemia 2 (BCL2, Bcl-2) family of proteins (Youle and Strasser, 2008). The pro-survival members {e.g. BCL2, BCL2L1 (Bcl-xL), MCL1 (Mcl-1), RFC1 (A1), and BCL2L2 (Bcl-w)} are essential for survival in a cell type-specific manner. A subfamily of pro-apoptotic members {multi-BHdomain subfamily-BAX, BAK1 (BAK), and possibly also BOK)}are critical for activation of the downstream events that result in cell death, while another sub-family {BH3-only proteins, including BCL2L11 (BIM), BBC3 (PUMA), BID, BAD, BMF, BIK, HRK, and PMAIP1 (NOXA)} initiate apoptosis signalling by activating BAX and BAK1protein molecules either through direct binding or, indirectly, through binding to pro-survival BCL2 family members, causing release of cytochrome-c and other apoptogenic factors from the mitochondria. Subsequently, this results in the formation of the apoptosome, which promotes activation of initiator and executioner proteins or caspases (*c*ysteine-*asp*artic prote*ases*). There are two types of apoptotic caspases: initiator (apical) caspases and effector (executioner) caspases. Initiator caspases (Caspase 2, 8, 9 and 10) cleave inactive pro-forms of effector caspases (Caspase 3, 6 and 7) thereby activating them to cleave other protein substrates within the cell and trigger the apoptotic process.

Bcl-2 family of Proteins

The B cell/lymphoma-2 family (Bcl-2) of proteins includes both, inhibitors (Bcl-2, Mcl-1, Bcl-xL, Bcl-w, amongst an assortment of others) and promoters (Bax, BAD, Bak and Bok among others) of apoptosis that govern mitochondrial outer membrane permeabilization (MOMP) and are evolutionarily related. There are a total of 25 genes in the Bcl-2 family known to date.

Bcl-2 family contributes to the checkpoints between cell surface and internal death signals, formation of apoptosome and activation of the caspase cascade (Sato *et al.*, 1994). Bcl-2 protein counteracts

Bax, and when Bax is in excess, cells execute a death command; but, when Bcl-2 dominates, the program is inhibited and cells survive. An expanded family of Bcl-2-related proteins share homology clustered within four conserved regions (Fig. 1) termed Bcl-2 homology 1through 4 (BH1, BH2, BH3 and BH4). These novel domains control the ability of these proteins to dimerize and function. An amphipathic á-helix, BH3, is of particular importance for the pro apoptotic family members (Korsmeyer, 1999) also called as the BH3-only proteins.

All pro-apoptotic and pro-survival (anti-apoptotic) proteins belong to the Bcl-2 family (Reed *et al.*, 1996). Anti-apoptotic proteins contain BH1 and BH2 domains, some of them contain an additional N-terminal BH4 domain (Bcl-2, Bcl-x(L), Bcl-w), which is also seen in some pro-apoptotic proteins like Bcl-x(S), Diva, Bok-L and Bok-S. Some anti-apoptotic protein such as Bcl-2 or Bcl-x (L) also contain BH3 domain.

All pro-apoptotic proteins contain a BH3 domain necessary for dimerization with other proteins of Bcl-2 family and crucial for their killing activity. Some of them also contain BH1 and BH2 domains (Bax, Bak).

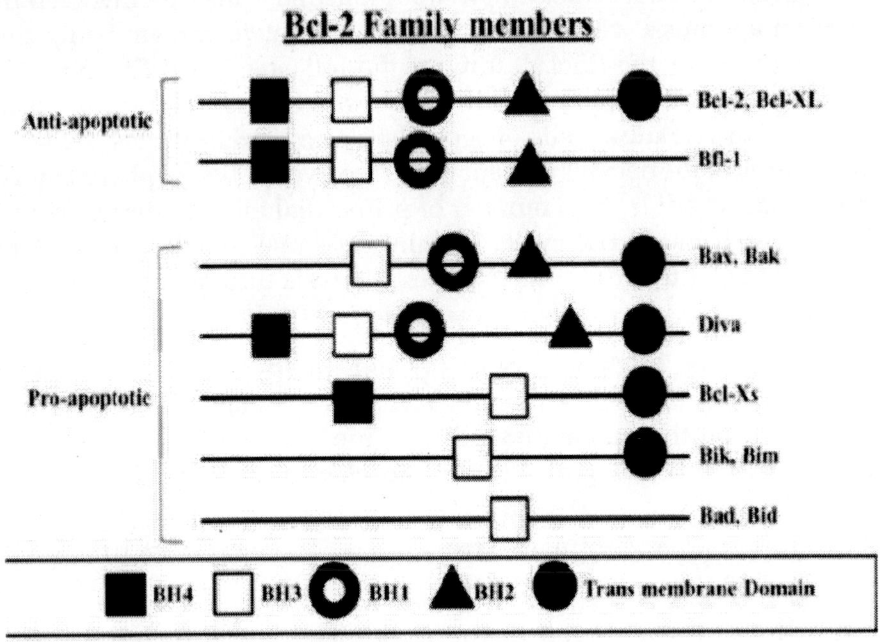

Fig. 1. Antiapoptotic and proapoptotic Bcl-2 family members (modified from Chao and Korsmeyer, 1998)

BH3-only family of proteins (Bim, Bid, BAD and others) contain only a single BH-domain. Various apoptotic stimuli induce expression and/or activation of specific BH3-only family members, which translocate to the mitochondria and initiate Bax/Bak-dependent apoptosis.

Ovarian Apoptosis

Cell death was first described in rabbit ovaries (Graaffian follicles), the phenomenon initially being called 'chromatolysis' (Hussein, 2005). Apoptosis is central to many aspects of the ovary. To date, apoptosis has been reported to be involved in oogenesis, folliculogenesis, oocyte loss/selection and atresia. Within the germ line, apoptosis may serve all of these functions depending on the stage of development, the nature of the extracellular environment, the status of intracellular metabolism, the integrity of the cell, and whether it is the male or female germ line under consideration (Aitkin *et al.*, 2011). In mammals, programmed cell death has been identified as the mechanism underlying the depletion of oocytes from the ovarian pool throughout life (Morita and Tilly, 1999; Tilly, 2001).

Several pro-survival and pro-apoptotic molecules are involved in ovarian apoptosis with the delicate balance between them being the determinant for the final destiny of the follicular cells. During fetal life, apoptosis is localized to the oocytes, whereas in adult life, it is detected in granulosa cells of secondary and antral follicles. At least two-thirds of the oocytes present in the reserve die by apoptosis before birth. During adult life, a number of primordial follicles start growing during each menstrual cycle. Usually only one follicle will ovulate and the fate of the rest of the follicles is atresia through apoptotic cell death.

Apoptosis in the ovary is carried out by several molecular pathways, of which Bcl-2 family, TNF, caspases and TGF-b proteins appear to be the major players. The molecules involved in these pathways can be categorized into four classes (Hussein, 2005):

i) Molecules that are involved in follicular survival, including Bcl-2, TGF-b, c-Kit, NOBOX, NTS, survivin, XIAP, AHR, BMP, GATA-4, SCF, integrin and GnRH

ii) Molecules involved in the follicular atresia, including Fas, caspases, TNF, TVB, Par-4, p53, prohibitin, c-Myc, interferon and ET

iii) Molecules involved in follicular selection/loss, including Bcl-2, Bax, FSH, inhibin, Fas ligand and caspases

iv) Molecules involved in luteogenesis, including Fas/Fas ligand, caspase 3, Bax, prohibitin, BMP ligands and receptors (BMPR receptors) and PGF2.

Studies in mice and humans have showed that death of primordial germ cells, oogonia and oocytes is mediated through Bcl-2 family of proteins (Ratts *et al.*, 1995, Rucker *et al.*,2000, Flaws *et al.*, 2001, Greenfeld *et al.*, 2007). Other Bcl-2 family members involved in ovarian apoptosis include Mcl-1, Bok (Bcl-2-related ovarian killer), Bod (Bcl-2-related ovarian death agonist) and Bad (Hussein, 2005). Gene over expression and knockout studies in mice have demonstrated that deregulation of the Bcl-2 regulated apoptosis pathway has a dramatic effect on the initial number of primordial follicles making up the ovarian reserve (Aitken *et al.*, 2011).

Expression of Bax has been observed to be upregulated in ovaries during follicular endowment and in cultured fetal oocytes undergoing apoptosis (De Felici *et al.*, 1999). Rucker *et al.* (2000) observed that if the anti-apoptotic protein Bcl-2L1 was deleted, the neonatal ovaries had a deficiency of oocytes apparently due to a failure to survive during embryonic life. Deletion (Ratts *et al.*, 1995) or overexpression (Flaws *et al.*, 2001) of Bcl-2 have been found to lead to either reduced oocyte endowment or enhanced oocyte endowment, respectively.

In granulosa cells of both, fetal and adult ovaries, Nandedkar and Dharma (2001) suggested that the expressed proteins Bcl-2 (pro survival), Bax (pro-apoptotic) and c-Myc were possibly involved in atresia. Van Nassauw *et al.* (1999) observed that Bcl-2 was mainly found in the developing follicles while Bax was mainly located in the atretic follicles.

Bcl-2 protein expression is found in all components of the human foetal ovaries (19–33 gestational weeks) to overcome extensive apoptotic activity (Abir *et al.*, 2002). This expression is related to gonadotrophin levels, where higher levels of gonadotrophin increase the expression of Bcl-2 and decrease the expression of Bax (Sugino *et al.*, 2000). Also, whereas Bcl-2/Bax ratio regulates apoptosis of the primordial follicle under SCF (survival molecule), Bax-mediated apoptosis in oocytes is mostly due to intrinsic meiotic checkpoints (De Felici *et al.*, 1999). Using Bax and Bcl-2 transcripts as markers, early apoptosis in the immature bovine oocytes has been found to be beneficial for developmental competence of the developing embryo at post fertilization, while none of the immature oocytes undergo late-stage apoptosis (Li *et al.*, 2008).

Select Apoptosis Modulator Proteins of Bcl-2 Family

i) The B cell/lymphoma-2 (Bcl-2) protein and *Bcl-2* gene

The Bcl-2protein is a pro-survival molecule identified through its involvement in B-cell lymphoma-2 and is encoded by the *Bcl*-2 gene.

Orthologs have been identified in numerous animals whose complete genome data are available. The two isoforms of Bcl-2, Isoform 1 and Isoform 2, exhibit similar fold but differ by two amino acids and in the ability of these isoforms to bind to the Bad and Bak proteins, as well as in the structural topology and electrostatic potential of the binding groove, suggesting differences in their anti-apoptotic activity (Petros *et al.*, 2001). It is a membrane-associated protein that resides in the nuclear envelope and mitochondria. It exerts its pro-survival functions by various mechanisms (MacManus and Linnik, 1997; Hussein, 2005) including, modulating the mitochondrial release of cytochrome c and the interaction of Apaf-1 with caspase- 9; binding to Bax; and blocking apoptosis induced by c-Myc.

Alternatively, Bcl-xL (long isoform) has stronger pro-survival effects than Bcl-2 itself. The expression of this protein protects cells from entering p53-mediated apoptosis (Boyd *et al.*, 1995). The anti-apoptotic Bcl-2 and Bcl-xL proteins inhibit cytochrome c release through the mitochondrial pore thus inhibiting activation of the cytoplasmic caspase cascade (Helmreich, 2001).

The pro - or anti-apoptotic activities of the *Bcl* - 2 family members are regulated not only at the transcriptional level, but also at the post-translational level, including phosphorylation, cleavage, translocation, and dimerization (Gross *et al.*, 1999). *Bcl-2* although important for regulating oocyte survival, yet appears to be expressed at low levels in human (Guillemin *et al.*, 2009) and mouse oocytes (Exley *et al.*, 1999). However, its pro-apoptotic homolog *Bax* appears to be consistently expressed in human (Jurisicova *et al.* 2003) and mouse oocytes (Exley *et al.* 1999), albeit with increased expression levels in oocytes of aged mice (Perez *et al.*, 2005).

ii) Bcl-2-associated X (Bax) protein and *Bax* gene

Bax {Bcl-2-associated X protein/Bcl-2-like protein 4 (BCL2L4)} encoded by the *Bax* gene is another pro-apoptotic Bcl-2 homologue that resides either in the cytoplasm or in the cell membrane and can antagonize the protective role of Bcl-2. The Bcl-2 family members form hetero-or homodimers and act as anti- or pro-apoptotic regulators that are involved in a wide variety of cellular activities (Fig. 2).

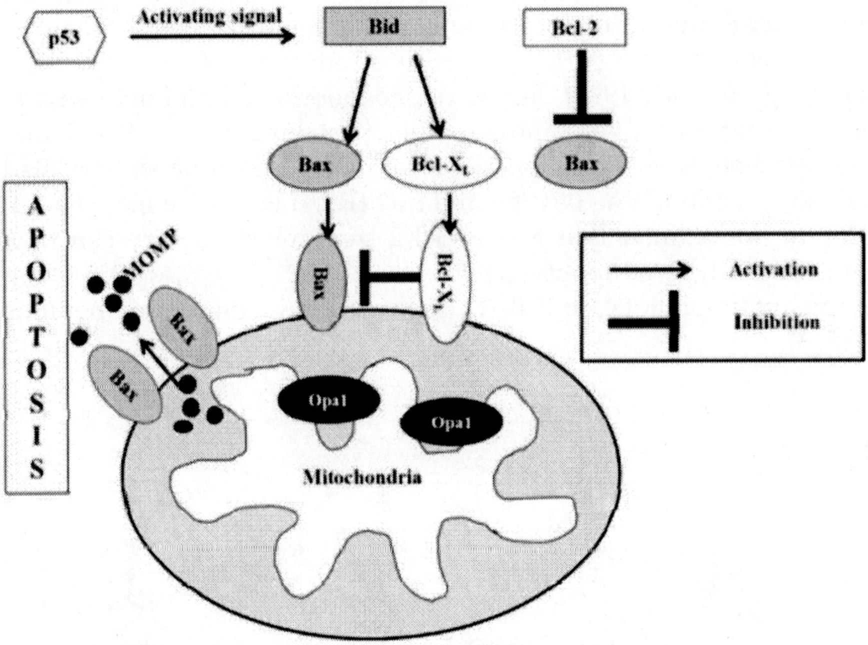

Fig. 2. Regulation of apoptosis by Bax and modulation by Bcl-2

Bax forms a heterodimer with Bcl-2, and functions as an apoptotic activator and have been reported to interact with, and increase the opening of, the mitochondrial voltage-dependent anion channel (VDAC), which leads to the loss in membrane potential and the release of cytochrome c (Shi *et al.*, 2003). There is also recent evidence that activated *BAX* and/or Bak form an oligomeric pore (Mitochondrial Apoptosis-Induced Channel or MAC) in the outer membrane (Buytaert *et al.*, 2006) resulting in the release of cytochrome-c and other pro-apoptotic factors from the mitochondria (mitochondrial outer membrane permeabilization), leading to activation of caspases. This direct role for *BAX* is common to all Bcl-2 member proteins containing the BH1, BH2 and BH3 domains. The expression of the *Bax* gene is regulated by the tumour suppressor P53 and has been shown to be involved in P53-mediated apoptosis. Multiple alternatively spliced transcript variants, which encode different isoforms, have been reported for the gene encoding the *Bax* gene.

Bcl-2-associated Death Promoter (Bad) Protein and Bad gene

Bad (Bcl-2-associated death promoter) is a member of the BH3-only subfamily of the Bcl-2 family. It does not contain a C-terminal trans-membrane domain for outer mitochondrial membrane and nuclear envelope targeting, unlike most other members of the Bcl-2 family (Hsu *et al.*, 1997). Bad is dephosphorylated and activated to form a heterodimer with anti-apoptotic proteins Bcl-2 and Bcl-xL and prevent them from stopping apoptosis. When Bad is phosphorylated by Akt/protein kinase B (triggered by PIP_3), it forms the Bad-(14-3-3) protein homodimer that leaves Bcl-2 free, which in turn can now inhibit Bax triggered apoptosis (Helmreich, 2001). Bad phosphorylation is thus anti-apoptotic, and BAD dephosphorylation is pro-apoptotic (Fig. 3).

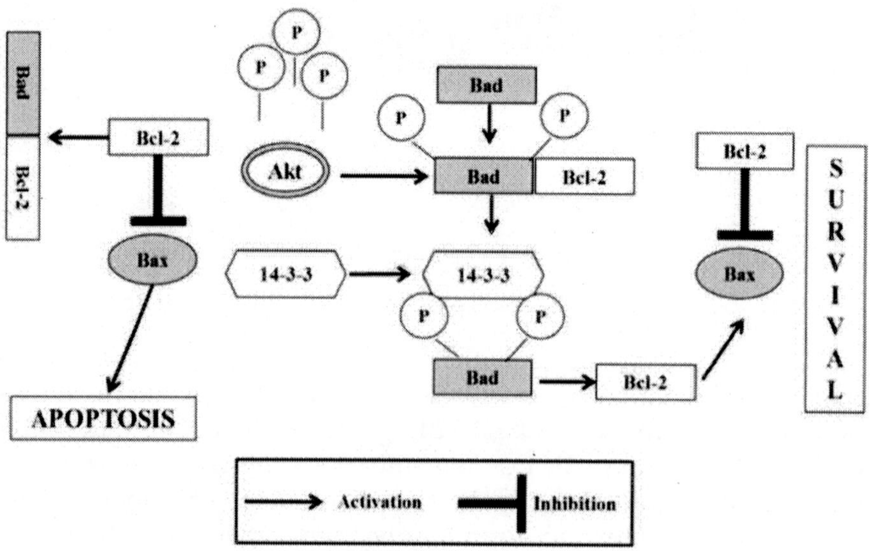

Fig. 3. Regulation of apoptosis by Bad and modulation by Bcl-2

Induction of Apoptosis by Heat Stress

Various pathological stimuli, such as radiation, environmental toxicants, oxidative stress, and heat shock can initiate apoptosis in mammalian oocytes (Roth and Hansen, 2004a). Studies have shown that the redox status of the cell, resulting from an accumulation of ROS and a decrease of antioxidant levels, is involved in inducing apoptotic cell death (Hockenbery *et al.*, 1993) and GSH presumably plays a critical role in regulating apoptosis by influencing the redox status (Boggs *et al.*, 1998).

Heat stress does have an overwhelming impact on the development of the oocyte. The negative effects may include alterations in the cytoplasmic and nuclear maturation, protein expression, membrane alterations, induction of apoptosis, premature aging and overall developmental competence (Maya-Soriano, 2012). Being less tolerant to thermal stress, changes in the cytoplasm are more pronounced than those of the nucleus (Wang *et al.*, 2008). Impaired intervention by either of the many counter-check mechanisms (anti-oxidants, heat shock proteins, etc.) may induce other biochemical and morphological changes, including progression to apoptosis- directly or through generation of free radicals, and thus, cellular injury. Many of the biological processes are intertwined and carefully synchronised, some regulators have been identified, some yet to be unravelled.

Thermal stress causes a fraction (approx. 15–30%) of maturing cattle oocytes to undergo apoptosis as determined by TUNEL labelling of the pronucleus (Roth and Hansen, 2004a; 2004b; 2005; Soto and Smith 2009). Inhibition of heat-shock-induced apoptosis with a caspase inhibitor (Roth and Hansen 2004a), sphingosine 1-phosphate (Roth and Hansen 2004b, 2005) or a BH4 peptide (Soto and Smith, 2009) reduced the effect of elevated culture temperature on oocyte competence for fertilization and subsequent development (Hansen, 2009).

Ahmed *et al.* (2016) recorded considerable reduction in development competence of bovine oocytes matured under elevated temperatures. Ultrastructural changes in *in vitro* matured bovine oocytes were found to be akin to those associated with apoptosis (Ahmed *et al.*, 2017). The expression profiles of anti-apoptotic protein Bcl-2 were also higher in heat-stressed surviving oocytes or when they were protected with antioxidant incorporation in the maturation media (Ahmed, 2014), on the other hand-proapoptotic proteins Bad and Bax were found to be elevated during apoptosis.

In the developing embryo, there are also evidences that ROS production by elevated temperatures lead to apoptosis. Yang *et al.*,

(1998) in a study on human embryos cultured in ambient oxygen environment concluded that there was a direct relationship between increased H_2O_2 concentration and apoptosis, and that ROS caused morphological changes, such as cytoplasmic condensation and apoptotic bodies demonstrable electron microscopically. In cattle induction of apoptosis by elevated temperature does not occur until the 8-16 cell stage at day 4 after insemination (Paula-Lopes and Hansen, 2002a). In another study, Paula-Lopes and Hansen (2002b) found that group II caspases mediate heat-induced apoptosis in bovine pre-implantation embryos, and that inhibition of these caspases instead had a detrimental effect on embryonic resistance to heat shock. The authors therefore suggested that apoptosis be viewed as an adaptive mechanism to allow embryonic survival and development following stress.

There have been many studies on the molecular signalling of cells in response to heat shock. The Mitogen associated protein kinase (MAPK) pathways is one proposed mechanism of cell signalling during cellular stresses, such as osmotic shock, arsenite, and heat shock (Moriguchi *et al.*, 1996). Other MAPK homologues or its subfamily of kinases, Jun kinase (JNK) and reactivated kinase (RK) or p38 (Rouse *et al.*, 1994), are stress-activated protein kinases (SAPKs), which relay heat shock and oxidative stress signals in mammalian cells.

Ju (2005) summarized that thermotolerance of the oocyte and the embryo may not simply correlate with synthesis of HSPs, and could be caused, at least in part, by heat shock-induced apoptosis and alterations of the chromatin and spindle microtubules. Another mechanism of apoptosis is the generation of heat-elevated free radicals in the oocyte or embryos that may contribute to their low developmental competence (Hansen *et al.*, 2001; Rivera and Hansen, 2001). Other factors, such as anti-oxidative defence system, uterine environment and circulating hormonal profile of the animal are also involved (Ju, 2005). In addition, heat shock may cause calcium ion elevation in the cell (Stevenson *et al.*, 1986) that leads to apoptosis of the oocytes and embryos probably through MAPK cascades (Ju, 2005).

Conclusion

It is thus evident that apoptosis plays a dual role for determining the fate of incompetent or inferior follicular cells as a part of the natural selection procedure. On the other hand, adverse situations including heat-stressors, free-radical insult and other unwarranted factors may induce the competent cells to undergo cell death. Exposure to heat stress due to elevated ambient temperature is often recognized as a major factor responsible for reduced fertility in farm animals. In the context of the present global scenario of climatic changes, heat stress induced by adverse elements can bring about increasing failures in reproduction and development competence of oocytes. As the molecular mechanisms are being unravelled and demystified, newer insights would help formulate and devise strategies to counter the harmful and deleterious effects of heat stress and reproductive failures.

References

1. Abir, R.; Orvieto, R.; Dicker, D.; Zukerman, Z.; Barnett, M. and Fisch, B. (2002). Preliminary studies on apoptosis in human fetal ovaries. *Fertil. Steril.*, **78**: 259-264.

2. Ahmed, J.A. (2014). Antioxidant Intervention during *in vitro* Maturation-Fertilization and Expression of Certain Apoptotic Genes in Heat Stress Induced Bovine Oocytes. PhD thesis. Assam Agricultural University, Guwahati, India.

3. Ahmed, J.A.; Dutta, D.J. and Nashiruddullah, N. (2016). Comparative efficacy of antioxidant retinol, melatonin, and zinc during *in vitro* maturation of bovine oocytes under induced heat stress. *Turk. J. Vet. Anim. Sci.*, **4**: 365-373.

4. Ahmed, J.A.; Nashiruddullah, N.; Dutta, D.; Biswas, R.K. and Borah, P. (2017). Cumulus cell expansion and ultrastructural changes in *in vitro* matured bovine oocytes under heat stress. *Iranian J. Vet. Res.*, 18:203-207

5. Aitken, R.J., Findlay, J.K.; Hutt, K.J. and Kerr, J.B. (2011). Apoptosis in the germ line. *Reprod.*, **141**: 139–150.

6. Boggs, S.E.; McCormick, T.S. and Lapetina, E.G. (1998). Glutathione levels determine apoptosis in macrophages. *Biochem. Biophys. Res. Commun.*, **247**: 229–233.

7. Boyd, J.M.; Gallo, G.J.; Elangovan, B.; Houghton, A.B.; Malstrom, S.; Avery, B.J.; Ebb, R.G.; Subramanian, T.; Chittenden, T. and Lutz, R.J. (1995). Bik, a novel death-inducing protein shares a distinct sequence motif with Bcl-2 family proteins and interacts with viral and cellular survival-promoting proteins. *Oncogene*, **11**: 1921–1928.

8. Buytaert, E.; Callewaert, G.; Vandenheede, J.R. and Agostinis, P. (2006). Deficiency in apoptotic effectors Bax and Bak reveals an autophagic cell death pathway initiated by photodamage to the endoplasmic reticulum. *Autophagy*, **2**(3): 238–240.

9. Chao, D.T. and Korsmeyer, S.J. (1998). BCL-2 family: regulators of cell death. *Annu. Rev. Immunol.*, **16**: 395–419.

10. De Felici, M.D.; Carlo, A.D.; Pesce, M.; Iona, S.; Farrace, M.G. and Piacentini, M. (1999). Bcl-2 and Bax regulation of apoptosis in germ cells during prenatal oogenesis in the mouse embryo. *Cell Death Differentiation*, **6**: 908–915.

11. Exley, G.E.; Tang, C.; McElhinny, A.S. and Warner, C.M. (1999). Expression of caspase and *BCL-2* apoptotic family members in mouse preimplantationembryos.*Biol.Reprod.*,**61:** 231–239.

12. Flaws, J.A.; Hirshfield, A.N.; Hewitt, J.A.; Babus, J.K. and Furth, P.A. (2001). Effect of Bcl-2 on the primordial follicle endowment in the mouse ovary. *Biol. Reprod.*, **64**: 1153–1159.

13. Greenfeld, C.R.; Pepling, M.E.; Babus, J.K.; Furth, P.A. and Flaws, J.A. (2007). BAX regulates follicular endowment in mice. *Reprod.*,**133**: 865–876.

14. Gross, A.; McDonnell, J.M. and Korsmeyer, S.J. (1999). *BCL-2* family members and the mitochondria in apoptosis. *Genes Dev.*, **13**:1899-911.

15. Guillemin, Y.; Lalle, P.; Gillet, G.; Guerin, J.F.; Hamamah, S. and Aouacheria, A. (2009). Oocytes and early embryos selectively express the survival factor BCL2L10. *J. Mol. Medicine.*, **87**: 923–940.

16. Hansen, P.J. (2009). Effects of heat stress on mammalian reproduction. *Phil. Trans. R. Soc. B.*, **364**: 3341–3350.

17. Hansen, P.J.; Drost, M.; Rivera, R.M.; Paula-Lopes, F.F.; Al-Katanani, Y.M.; Krininger, C.E. III, Chase, C.C. Jr. (2001). Adverse impact of heat stress on embryo production: causes and strategies for mitigation. A review. *Theriogenology*, **55**: 91-103.

18. Helmreich, E.J.M. (2001). The Biochemistry of Cell Signalling. Oxford University Press, pp. 238-243.

19. Hockenbery, D.M.; Oltvai, Z.N.; Yin, X.M.; Milliman, C.L. and Korsmeyer, S.J. (1993). Bcl-2 functions in an antioxidant pathway to prevent apoptosis. *Cell*, **75**: 241–251.

20. Hsu, S.Y.; Kaipia, A.; Zhu, L. and Hsueh, A.J.W. (1997). Interference of BAD (Bcl-xL/Bcl-2-Associated Death Promoter)-induced apoptosis in mammalian cells by 14–3-3 isoforms and P11. *Mol. Endocrinol.*, **11**(12): 1858–1867.

21. Hussein, M.R. (2005). Apoptosis in the ovary: molecular mechanisms. *Human Reprod. Update*, **11**(2): 162–178.

22. Ju, J.C. (2005). Cellular responses of oocytes and embryos under thermal stress: hints to molecular signalling. *Anim. Reprod.*, **2**(2): 79-90.

23. Jurisicova, A.; Antenos, M.; Varmuza, S.; Tilly, J.L.and Casper, R.F. (2003). Expression of apoptosis-related genes during human preimplantation embryo development: potential roles for the Harakiri gene product and caspase-3 in blastomere fragmentation. *Mol. Hum. Reprod.*,**9**:133–141.

24. Kerr, J.F.; Wyllie, A.H. and Currie, A.R. (1972). Apoptosis: a basic biological phenomenon with wide-ranging implications in tissue kinetics. *Brit. J. Cancer*, **26**: 239–257.

25. Korsmeyer, S.J. (1999). BCL-2 gene family and the regulation of programmed cell death. *Cancer Res.*, **59**(Suppl.): 1693s-1700s.

26. Li, H.J.; Liu, D.J.; Cang, M.; Wang, L.M.; Jin, M.Z.; Ma, Y.Z. and Shorgan, B. (2008). Early apoptosis is associated with improved developmental potential in bovine oocytes. *Anim. Reprod. Sci.*, **114**(1-3): 89-98.

27. MacManus, J.P. and Linnik, M.D. (1997). Gene expression induced by cerebral ischemia: an apoptotic perspective. *J. Cerebral Blood Flow Metabolism*, **17**: 815–832.

28. Maya-Soriano, M.J. (2012). Heat Stress and Antioxidant Agents: Effects on Gamete Development. PhD Dissertation, UniverstatAutonoma de Barcelona, Spain.

29. Moriguchi, T.; Gotoh, Y. and Nishida, E. (1996). Roles of the MAP kinase cascades in vertebrates. *Adv. Pharmacol.*, **36**: 121-137.

30. Morita, Y. and Tilly, J.L. (1999). Oocyte apoptosis: like sand through an hourglass. *Develop. Biol.*, **213**:1–17.

31. Nandedkar, T.D. and Dharma, S.J. (2001). Expression of bcl(xs) and c-myc in atretic follicles of mouse ovary. *Reprod. Biomed. Online*, **3**: 221–225.

32. Paula-Lopes, F.F. and Hansen, P.J. (2002a). Heat-shock induced apoptosis in bovine preimplantation embryos is a developmentally-regulated phenomenon. *BiolReprod.*, **66**:1169–1177.

33. Paula-Lopes, F.F. and Hansen, P.J. (2002b). Apoptosis is an adaptive response in bovine preimplantation embryos that facilitates survival after heat shock. *Biochem. Biophys. Res. Commun.*, **295**:37–42.

34. Perez, G.I.; Jurisicova, A.; Matikainen, T.; Moriyama, T.; Kim, M.R.; Takai, Y.; Pru, J.K.; Kolesnick, R.N. and Tilly, J.L. (2005). A central role for ceramide in the age related acceleration of apoptosis in the female germline. *FASEB J.*, **19**: 860–862.

35. Petros, A.M.;Medek, A.; Nettesheim, D.G.; Kim, D.H.; Yoon, H.S.; Swift, K.; Matayoshi, E.D.; Oltersdorf, T. and Fesik, S.W. (2001). Solution structure of the antiapoptotic protein Bcl-2. *Proc. Natl. Acad. Sci. U.S.A.*, **98**(6): 3012–3017.

36. Ratts, V.S.; Flaws, J.A.; Kolp, R.; Sorenson, C.M. and Tilly, J.L. (1995). Ablation of Bcl-2 gene expression decreases the numbers of oocytes and primordial follicles established in the post-natal female mouse gonad. *Endocrinol.*,**136**: 3665–3668.

37. Reed, J.C.; Zha, H.; Aime-Sempe, C.; Takayama, S. and Wang, H.G. (1996). Structure-function analysis of Bcl-2 family proteins. Regulators of programmed cell death. *Adv. Exp. Med. Biol.*, **406**: 99–112.

38. Rivera, R.M. and Hansen, P.J. (2001). Development of cultured bovine embryos after exposure to high temperatures in physiological range. *Reprod.*,**121**: 107-115.

39. Roth, Z. and Hansen, P.J. (2004a). Involvement of apoptosis in disruption of developmental competence of bovine oocytes by heat shock during maturation. *Biol. Reprod.*, **71**: 1898–1906.

40. Roth, Z. and Hansen, P.J. (2004b). Sphingosine 1-phosphate protects bovine oocytes from heat shock during maturation. *Biol. Reprod.*, **71**: 2072–2078.

41. Roth, Z. and Hansen, P.J. (2005). Disruption of nuclear maturation and rearrangement of cytoskeletal elements in bovine oocytes exposed to heat shock during maturation. *Reprod.*,**129**: 235-244.

42. Rouse, J.; Cohen, P.; Trigon, S.; Morange, M.; Alonso-Llamazares, A.; Zamanillo, D.; Hunt, T. and Nebreda, A.R. (1994). A novel kinase cascade triggered by chemical stress and heat shock which stimulates MAP kinase activated protein kinase-2 and phosphorylation of the small heat shock proteins. *Cell*, **78**: 1027-1037.

43. Rucker, E.B. III; Dierisseau, P.; Wagner, K.U.; Garrett, L.; Wynshaw-Boris, A.; Flaws, J.A. and Hennighausen, L. (2000). Bcl-x and Bax regulate mouse primordial germ cell survival and apoptosis during embryogenesis. *Mol. Endocrinol.*, **14**: 1038–1052.

44. Sato, T.; Hanada, M.;Bodrug, S.;Irie, S.; Iwama, N,; Boise, L.H.; Thompson, C.B.; Golemis, E.; Fong, L. and Wang, H.G. (1994). Interactions among members of the Bcl-2 protein family analyzed with a yeast two-hybrid system. *Proc. Natl. Acad. Sci. U.S.A.*, **91**:9238–9242.

45. Shi, Y.; Chen, J.; Weng, C.; Chen, R.; Zheng, Y.; Chen, Q. and Tang, H. (2003). Identification of the protein-protein contact site and interaction mode of human VDAC1 with Bcl-2 family proteins. *Biochem. Biophys. Res. Commun.*, **305**(4): 989–996.

46. Soto, P. and Smith, L.C. (2009). BH4 peptide derived from Bcl-xL and Bax-inhibitor peptide suppresses apoptotic mitochondrial changes in heat stressed bovine oocytes. *Mol. Reprod. Develop.*,**76**: 637-646.

47. Stevenson, M.A.; Calderwood, S.K. and Hahn, G.M. (1986). Rapid increases in inositol trisphosphate and intracellular Ca^{2+} after heat shock. *Biochem. Biophys. Res. Comm.*, **137**: 826-833.

48. Sugino, N.; Suzuki, T.; Kashida, S.; Karube, A.; Takiguchi, S. and Kato, H. (2000). Expression of Bcl-2 and Bax in the human corpus luteum during the menstrual cycle and in early pregnancy: regulation by human chorionic gonadotropin. *J. Clin. Endocrinol. Metabol.*,**85**: 4379–4386.

49. Tilly, J.L. (2001). Commuting the death sentence: how oocyte strive to survive. *Nature Rev. Mol. Cell Biol.*, **2**:838–848.

50. Van Nassauw, L.; Tao, L. and Harrisson, F. (1999). Distribution of apoptosis related proteins in the quail ovary during folliculogenesis: BCL-2, BAX and CPP32. *ActaHistochem.*,**101**: 103–112.

51. Wang, J.Z.; Sui, H.S.; Miao, D.Q.; Liu, N.; Zhou, P. Ge, L. and Tan, J.H. (2008). Effects of stress during *in vitro* maturation of cytoplasmic versus nuclear components of mouse oocytes. *Reprod.*,**137**: 1-10.

52. Yang, H.W.; Hwang, K.J.; Kwon, H.C.; Kim, H.S.; Choi, K.W. and Oh, K.S. (1998). Detection of reactive oxygen species (ROS) and apoptosis in human fragmented embryos. *Human Reprod.*,**13**(4): 998–1002.

53. Youle, R.J. and Strasser, A. (2008). The BCL-2 protein family: opposing activities that mediate cell death. *Nature Rev. Mol. Cell Biol.*, **9**: 47–59.

□□□

Chapter 8

In vitro Maturation of Mammalian Oocytes

SUDHIR KUMAR*, UTSAV SHARMA AND SHARAD KUMAR

Division of Veterinary Gynaecology and Obstetrics, Faculty of Veterinary Sciences and Animal Husbandry, SKUAST-J, R. S. Pura, Jammu-181102 (J&K), India, *E-mail : sudhir_skuast@yahoo.com

1. Introduction

In vitro maturation (IVM) of oocytes is one of the essential and foremost steps in the *in vitro* fertilization (IVF) process. A number of researchers have studied different aspects of IVM in mammalian oocytes (Roa *et al.*, 2002; Kharche *et al.*, 2005). In most of the studies, the basic medium is supplemented with hormones and different concentrations of serum. The maturation mediums with the selection of protein supplements and hormones for IVM play an important role in subsequent IVF and *in vitro* development (Pawshe *et al.*, 1996). *In vitro* maturation of large number of oocytes provides an excellent opportunity for cheap and abundant embryo for carrying out basic research and for the application of emerging biotechnologies like cloning and transgenic. *In vitro* embryo production (IVEP) using abattoir derived ovaries as a source of oocytes is of a vast importance not only for the low cost mass production of bovine embryos for agriculture purposes but also as a research tool for improving its genetic merits at high rate as well as understanding this animal embryology that help improving its population (Mayes, 2002; Sagirkaya *et al.*, 2004: Camargo *et al.*, 2006). IVM of mammalian oocytes is affected by several factors, such as transport time and temperature from the slaughter- house to the laboratory, follicle size on the ovary, developmental stage of oocyte, oocyte diameter, composition of media, hormones and serum.

2. Phases of Oocyte Maturation

Oocyte maturation is a complex long cellular process involving both meiotic cycle progression (from diplotene to Metaphase-II) and cytoplasmic events reprogramming to enable the oocyte to attain its developmental competence to be fertilized and undergo embryogenesis (Shamsuddin, 1993; Eppig, 1996). During folliculogenesis, the oocyte grow, matured and attained the competence to be fertilized and undergo normal embryogenesis while, *in vitro* matured oocytes should bypass what was called the oocyte capacitation (the ultra-structural modifications took place in the oocyte of dominant follicles before the LH peak) (Hyttel *et al.*, 1997) and other substantial changes that ordinary took place *in vivo* under the influence of LH and the follicular environment (Motlik and Fulka, 1981), which permit the oocytes to attain its full developmental competence (Hyttel *et al.*, 1997) could be divided into two categories, those involved in the resumption and completion of the first meiotic division referred to as nuclear maturation and those occurring in the cytoplasm referred as cytoplasmic maturation (Eppig, 1996).

2.1 Nuclear Maturation

Meiosis, a Greek word meaning reduction, is defined as the unique cell division, that produces gametes or two cell divisions with no intervening with DNA replication resulting in halving of the chromosome complement (Mayes, 2002). Thus, the main aim of meiosis was to create haploid gametes and to allow genetic recombination resulting in generation of genetically unique gametes (Grondahl, 2008).

The mammalian oocytes begin meiosis during fetal life but don't complete meiosis-I until ovulation and meiosis-II was only completed upon fertilization (Hunt and Hassold, 2002). When meiosis resume, the arrested oocytes at the prophase I displaying a visible nucleus referred to as germinal vesicle (GV) (Grondahl, 2008) and this GV undergo germinal vesicle breakdown (GVBD) (i.e. dissolution of the nuclear envelope) (Mayes, 2002; Grondahl, 2008). The nucleolus disappears rapidly after coming in contact with the cytoplasm and chromatin condenses in what was called diakinesis phase (Mayes, 2002). During diakinesis, the nuclear membrane starts to fold, the nuclear pores disappear, then the nuclear membrane fragments before disappearing rapidly to leave only small sacs with double walls (Szollosi *et al.*, 1972; Kubelka *et al.*, 1988). Where then, the kinetochores appear and the microtubules pull the homologues chromosomes that were paired aligning on the meiotic spindle at metaphase-I (M-I) (Grondahl, 2008). This phase was accompanied by dramatic decrease of mRNA transcription and characteristic alterations in the protein synthesis (Tomek *et al.*, 2002). During *in vitro* maturation RNA synthesis strongly decreased because the condensed DNA present in oocytes from GVBD stage was practically disable for transcription, although, the translation increased only from GV to GVBD then decreased up to metaphase-II (Smiljakoviae and Tomek, 2006). After M-I phase the oocytes should pass through short anaphase I (i.e. migration of the chromosomes to their respective poles) and telophase-I (i.e. the chromosomes found at each pole are surrounded by a nuclear membrane). The oocytes become arrested at metaphase-I are referred to as 'partially competent' to undergo nuclear maturation (Eppig, 1996). Separation was completed, when metaphase-II (M-II) occurred, recognizable by the presence of 1st polar body (PB) (Grondahl, 2008, Marteil *et al.*, 2009). Now the oocyte remains arrested at the metaphase-II stage until fertilization (Kubelka *et al.*, 1988). Meiosis was completed following successful fertilization and could be confirmed by the presence of the 2nd PB.

2.2 Cytoplasmic Maturation

The endpoint of *in vivo* maturation was the release of a mature metaphase-II oocyte from the follicle, which upon sperm penetration, activation and genomic activation could support normal embryonic and fetal development to term and the birth of live offspring. On the other hand, the immature mammalian oocytes recovered from follicles were able to undergo spontaneous hormone independent resumption and completion of meiosis but they didn't appear to have full developmental competence under common *in vitro* maturation conditions as that evidenced by low morula and blastocyst rates of development (Moor and Trounson, 1977). The main reason for this incompetence was attributed to the deficient cytoplasmic maturation to enhance complete functional maturation of cow COCs *in vitro* (Totey *et al.*, 1993).

Cytoplasmic maturation could be defined as the unity of metabolic, molecular and ultra structural processes that modifying the oocyte cytoplasm for normal fertilization (Funahashi, 1998; Knobil and Neill, 1988) and acquisition of developmental competence (Hyttel *et al.*, 1986; Duranthon and Renard, 2001). It includes a wide array of synthesis for oocyte-specific developmentally regulated protein, relocation of cytoplasmic organelles and alteration to membrane transport system in the oocyte (Brevini-Gandolfi and Gandolfi, 2001; Watson, 2007). Furthermore, post-transcriptional modifications of mRNAs, proteins translation, post translational modification of proteins, substrates and nutrients that were accumulated during oogenesis and required to achieve oocyte developmental competence that fosters embryonic developmental competence (Levesque and Sirard, 1995; Watson, 2007). Moreover, ultra structural modification of the Golgi complex, accumulation of ribosomes and increase in lattice like structures (Kruip, *et al.*, 1983; Knobil and Neill, 1988).

Some elements of cytoplasmic maturation could be visualized (Knobil and Neill, 1988) whereas; many other elements were molecular and very challenging to visualize (Fulka *et al.*, 1998). For that, the cytoplasmic maturation was often divided into three major processes: organelle redistribution, cytoskeleton dynamics and molecular maturation (Ferreira *et al.*, 2009) and it could be used indirectly and retroactively to assess the ability of the mature oocyte to undergo normal fertilization, cleavage and blastocyst development. Failure to complete cytoplasmic maturation could block the development at fertilization, embryonic genome activation, blastocyst formation or even post implantation (Fuhrer *et al.*, 1989). Other indirect morphological parameters that could be taken into account to evaluate the cytoplasmic maturation were cumulus cell expansion, extrusion of the 1st PB and an increased perivitelline space (Kruip *et al.*, 1983).

In general, nuclear maturation was viewed only morphologically and for this reason it might be not consider as an absolute indicator for the normality after IVM, while, cytoplasmic maturation provides unequivocal information about the success of oocyte maturation. Ultimately, the quality and completeness of cytoplasmic maturation played an important role in the development of oocyte competence.

3. Various Factors Affecting *in vitro* Maturation of Mammalian Oocytes

3.1 Quality of Oocytes

Naturally, the oocyte quality is determined by the oocyte's ability to mature, be fertilized and give rise to normal offspring (Duranthon and Renard, 2001; Hussein *et al.*, 2006). The quality of the oocyte is also related to the oocyte's follicular environment (Camargo *et al.*, 2006), as well as several factors: such as age of the donor animal, stage of follicular development and the media used for maturing the oocytes. Cumulus investment morphology and the microscopic aspect of the ooplasm are generally considered as the two main parameters to assess the quality of the cumulus oocyte complex (COC) (De Loose *et al.*, 1989). The criteria employed by various scientists for selection of oocytes for IVM include the presence of a multilayer compact cumulus oophorus and homogeneous cytoplasm (Wurth *et al.*, 1992; De Wit *et al.*, 2000).

3.2 Presence of Cumulus Cells

Selection of bovine oocytes for IVM was performed on the basis of visual assessment for the morphological features (Leibfried and First, 1979). Cumulus cells establish intimate contacts together as well as with the oocyte to allow cell communication through gap junctions, which were necessary for efficient maturation of the oocyte (Van Soom, *et al.*, 2002). It had been reported that, the surrounding cumulus cells had a n essential role not only in nuclear maturation but also in cytoplasmic maturation, which was needed for male pronuclear formation (Chian *et al.*, 1994). In mouse, even if cumulus cells were not essential for normal oocyte fertilization (Schroeder and Eppig, 1984), their presence during meiotic maturation (in particular the maintenance of efficient gap junctions) could influence the oocyte competence to undergo normal fertilization and the acquisition of the capacity to transform the sperm nucleus into male pronucleus. It was interesting to know that when the granulosa cells differentiated into cumulus cells they produced a factor(s), which via paracrine signals could induce nuclear and cytoplasmic maturation in the oocytes derived from early antral or preovulatory follicles (Cecconi *et al.*, 1996). Moreover, it had been reported that the secretory products of cumulus cells had fundamental effects on the oocyte developmental competence. de Loose *et al.* (1991) described that the presence of an intact complement of cumulus cells surrounding the oocyte with a homogenous appearance of the ooplasm were the best predictive morphological criteria of immature oocyte ability to undergo maturation and high embryonic development. Upon that, when oocytes exhibiting cumulus oocyte complexes (COCs) with complete and compact cumulus investment were selected an average of 30 to 40% of them will eventually develop to the morula and blastocysts stages (Gordon, 1990).

3.3 Size of Ovarian Follicles

Generally oocytes are selected for IVM using the criteria like follicle size, cytoplasmic appearance, the appearance and number of cumulus cells around the oocytes (COC's). Cumulus expansion can importantly be used to microscopically assess the *in vitro* maturation rate of oocytes (Gupta *et al.*, 2005) and also Lonergan *et al.* (1994) and Yang *et al.* (1998) showed a relationship between follicle size and oocyte quality. It has been observed that follicular size profoundly influences the quality of the oocyte obtained during ovulation and the quality of embryo obtained (Sirard *et al.*, 2006). Follicle size, thus, affects the oocyte quality, potentially involving mRNA or protein reserves as factors involved in determining the oocyte competence (Krisher, 2004). At growth phase time, oocytes increase in diameter to more than 120 micron meter (μm). Researchers have demonstrated that oocytes with a diameter of less than 110 μm may still be in the growth phase which are less capable of developing after fertilization and results with lower rates of blastocyst formation. Such small oocytes are also prone to undergo certain chromosome alterations during maturation, which impairs further development (Lechniak, *et al.*, 2002).

Ovarian follicular size and oocyte diameter relationship exists and influences in meiotic progression in sheep (Shirazi, and Sadeghi, 2007). Follicle size as well as number of follicles on the ovarian surface plays an important role in embryonic development. Sheep ovaries with eight or more follicles on the surface have been shown to yield higher percentages of cleavage and blastocyst rates (94% and 52.4%, respectively), compared to 57% and 30.2% attained from ovaries having 4 or less follicles on the ovarian surface (Cognie, *et al.*,1995). In buffalo, Yousaf and Chohan (2003) found poor *in vitro* maturation rates (32% and 32.7%) to metaphase-II stage for oocytes isolated from 2 to <3 and from 3 to <3 mm follicles, respectively, whereas significantly ($P<0.05$) more oocytes from 4 to<6 and from 6 to <8 mm follicles reached M II (67.1% and 79.1, respectively). In contrary, Leibfried and First (1979) and Crister *et al.* (1986) found no difference in nuclear maturation and fertilization, when 1 to 5 mm follicles were cultured *in vitro*, but there were differences in the embryonic development.

3.4 Status of Ovary

Interactions occur among corpus luteum (CL) bearing ovaries, seasons, physiological status and feeding system. It has been stated that buffalo ovaries bearing CL had significantly ($P<0.05$) lower mean number of oocytes following aspiration (Amer *et al.*, 2008). Kumar *et al.* (1997) also recorded a low average yield from ovaries bearing CL (4.08) than that non-bearing CL (6.55). They demonstrated that this might be the result of a major portion of the ovary being occupied by the lutein cells, thereby restricting. However, Abdoon and Kandil (2001) found that number of surface ovarian follicles were significantly ($P<0.05$) higher on ovaries bearing CL than those non-bearing CL. On the other hand, Das *et al.* (1996) and Boediono *et al.* (1995) found a similar number of follicles and oocytes on ovaries with or without CL (3.55 and 2.68 vs.2.7/ovary, respectively). In bovine, Varisanga *et al.* (1998) found that oocyte yield per ovary from ovaries bearing CL was significantly higher ($P<0.01$) than ovaries without CL. Similar trend was reported by Dode *et al.* (2001), who found a higher number of oocytes from pregnant than non-pregnant cow ovaries.

3.5 Methods of Oocytes Recovery

Many methods for oocytes recovery had been described in domestic animals these methods were: dissection of the ovarian follicles, aspiration, slicing and puncture of visible surface follicles. By aspiration method the needles used as well as the aspiration vacuum were important factors in determining the number and quality of the oocytes, these parameters should be established for each species, where in cow, good results obtained with 18 gauge needle connected to a 3 cm Hg vacuum (Mermillod *et al.*, 2006). The oocytes recovered by aspiration method represent only 43.2% of the entire number of oocytes. This low recovery rate might be due to difficulties in separating the cumulus oophorus (Katska, 1984.). El-Gaafary and Abdel-Ghaffar (1994) showed that significantly more oocytes were recovered per ovary by dissection than aspiration. Das *et al.* (1996) demonstrated that slicing was a simple and effective method for collecting a high quality buffalo oocytes yield for *in vitro* culture, where the success rate was 5.7 oocytes per ovary. Even though, a significantly lower rate of oocytes reaching the metaphase-II stage was observed when using slicing techniques; this lower maturation rate might be due to more preantral oocytes collected (Wang *et al.*, 2007). On contrary, Pawshe *et al.* (1996) and Martino *et al.* (1994) noticed that there was non-significant difference in the blastocyst developmental rate between aspiration and slicing methods depending upon the culture system. Additionally, Carolan *et al.* (1993) found that, oocytes recovery by slicing rather than aspiration method can result in marked increase in blastocysts yield after IVM/IVF/IVC.

3.6 Media Additives

The culture medium, protein supplements and hormones for IVM play an important role in the subsequent maturation rate and embryonic development following IVF (Bavister *et al.*, 1992). Various culture media, such as TCM-199, minimum essential medium (MEM) and Ham's F-10 have been used for *in vitro* maturation of oocytes. TCM-199 is the most widely used and the beneficial effect on IVM of animal oocytes may be related to some factors in its composition such as essential amino acids and glutamine that stimulate DNA and RNA synthesis and enhance cell division (Pawshe *et al.*, 1996; Gordon, 2003).

Serum provides beneficial factors to the culture medium, including energy substrates, amino acids and vitamins. There may be specific effects of serum component possibly growth factors on oocyte maturation that are manifested as improved embryo development following IVF (Eppig *et al.*, 1992). Also, Downs *et al.* (1986) suggested that it may be important to include serum in the *in vitro* maturation medium to prevent hardening of zona pellucida, which could adversely affect fertilization. In addition to, Schroeder *et al.* (1990) observed that fetuin, a major glycoprotein constituent of fetal calf serum, can prevent hardening of zona pellucida during *in vitro* maturation, as it acts by preventing the action of proteolytic enzymes originating from precociously released cortical granules and improve the fertilization capacity of oocytes. Furthermore, serum added to the oocyte medium provides a source of albumin that balances the osmolarity (Thompson, 2000). There are different sources for supplemented sera such as fetal calf serum, oestrus buffalo serum, steer serum and superovulated buffalo serum.

Addition of hormones, such as follicle stimulating hormones, (FSH) pregnant mare serum gonadotrophin (PMSG), luteinizing hormone (LH) and estradiol to culture media has been made to improve the developmental competence of *in vitro* matured oocytes. In many species, gonadotropins have been found to stimulate cumulus cells to synthesize molecules able to drive germinal vesicle breakdown GVBD as meiosis activating sterols (Tsafriri *et al.*, 2005). Estradiol has been found to improve the completion of maturational changes and also to support the synthesis of presumed male pronuclear growth factor

(Fukui and Ono, 1989). The supplementation of maturation media with eduine chorionic gonado tropin (eCG) resulted in a higher *in vitro* maturation rate of buffalo oocytes than FSH (Hegab *et al.*, 2009). In addition, Alok *et al.* (2010) showed that FSH is essential for cumulus cell expansion and maturation of oocytes *in vitro* as FSH enhances the expansion of cumulus cells surrounding the oocytes, which in turn enhances sperm capacitation and the fertilization process.

3.7 Seasonal Variations

In general, the reproductive traits of animals are affected by climatic changes. Some degree of seasonal variation in breeding efficiency is usual with most of the domestic animals. Primarily, ambient temperature and relative humidity showed a direct effect on breeding efficiency (Roy *et al.*, 1968). Buffaloes subjected to heat stress yield fewer good quality oocytes than their unstressed counterparts (Zoheir *et al.*, 2007). There is relationship between season, quality of oocytes, cumulus cell expansion, maturation and developmental rates of *in vitro* maturation of oocytes (Zoheir *et al.*, 2007; El-Naby *et al.*, 2013). Leibfried-Rutledge *et al.* (1989) reported that high ambient temperature and humidity have deleterious effect on oocyte capability for maturation and fertilization *in vitro*. Moreover, Zeron *et al.* (2001) mentioned that the heat stress can alter phospholipids composition of oocytes. While, Nandi *et al.* (2001 stated that the external environmental conditions did not affect the fertilization, if the aspirated oocytes successfully completed maturation. In contrast, Kadoom (1995) recorded that the quality of oocytes was increased in summer season.

3.8 Time of Oocyte Maturation

Oocytes remained in the germinal vesicle (GV) stage from the onset to 6 to 8 h of culture. The germinal vesicle breakdown (GVBD) occurred between 7 to 9 h and the metaphase-I became established within 12 to 18 h. Lastly most oocytes reach the metaphase-II stage after 27 h (at 38.5°C) (Motlagh *et al.*, 2008). Most appropriate maturation period in both, cattle and buffaloes is 24 h. Gasparrini *et al.* (2007) reported that the attainment of the MII stage commenced after 18 h maturation but the majority of oocytes completed nuclear maturation between 21 and 24 h. In addition to, Nandi *et al.* (2002) observed that cumulus expansion and extrusion of 1st polar body in buffalo oocytes commence at 16 to 17 h post maturation to reach the maximum levels at 22 to 24 h. Other researchers have also reported that the highest proportion of MII oocytes occurs after 24 h of IVM in the same species (Singh and Majumdar 1992; Yadav *et al.*, 1997). Large variations in the timing of the oocyte maturation process *in vitro* have also been reported.

On conclusion, oocyte maturation is a complex process that is affected by many factors starting from its recovery process and ending by its culture. So, a great attention should be paid to all of these preceding factors to ensure efficient oocyte with high developmental competence. The investigations must be directed towards the various other factors affecting oocyte quality and *in vitro* maturation of mammalian oocytes.

References

Abdoon, A.S.S. and Kandil, O.M. 2001. Factor affecting number of surface ovarian follicles and oocytes yield and quality in Egyptian buffaloes. *Reprod. Nutr. Dev.*, 41: 71-77.

Alok, P., Gupta S.C. and Neelam, G. 2010. Effect of FSH and LH hormones on oocyte maturation of buffalo and gene expression analysis of their receptors and Cx43 in maturing oocytes. *Zygote*, 18(3): 231-234.

Amer, H.A., Hegab A.O. and Zaabal, S.M. 2008. Effects of ovarian morphology on oocyte quantity and quality, granulosa cells, *in vitro* maturation and steroid hormone production in buffaloes. *Anim. Reprod.* 5: 55-62

Bavister, B.D., Rose-Hellekant T.A. and Pinyopummintr, 1992. Development of *in vitro* matured/*in vitro* fertilized bovine embryos into morulae and blastocysts in defined culture media. *Theriogenology*, 37: 127-146.

Boediono, A., R. Rajamahendran, S. Saha, Sumantri C. and Suzuki, T. 1995. Effect of the presence of a CL in the ovary on oocyte number, cleavage rate and blastocyst production *in vitro* in cattle. *Theriogenology*, 43: 169.

Brevini-Gandolfi, T.A.L. and Gandolfi, F. 2001. The maternal legacy to the embryo: Cytoplasmic components and their effects on early development. *Theriogenology*, 55: 1255-1276.

Camargo, L.S.A., Viana J.H.M., Sa, W.F., Ferreira, A.M., Ramos, A.A. and Vale Filho, V.R. 2006. Factors influencing *in vitro* embryo production. *Anim Reprod*, **3**(1): 19-28.

Carolan, C., Monaghan, P., Gallagher, M. and Gordon, I. 1993. Developmental capacity of unselected bovine oocytes recovered from individual pairs of ovaries by surface dissection. *Proce. 9th Congress of the European Embryo Transfer Association (Lyon):* pp. 180.

Cecconi, S., Aurizio R. D. and Colonna, R. 1996. Role of antral follicle development and cumulus cells on *in vitro* fertilization of mouse oocytes. *J. Reprod Fertil*, 107: 207-214.

Chian, R.C., Niwa K.and Sirard, M.A. 1994. Effects of cumulus cell on male pronuclear formation and subsequent early development of bovine oocytes *in vitro*. *Theriogenology*, 41: 1499-1508.

Cognie, Y., Poulin, N. Pisselet C. and Monniaux, D. 1995. Effect of atresia on the ability of follicular fluid to support developmental competence of sheep oocytes *in vitro*. *Theriogenology*, 43(1): 188-188.

Crister, E.S., Leibfried-Rutledge, M.L. Eyestone, W.H. Northey D.L. and First, N.L. 1986. Acquisition of developmental competence during maturation *in vitro*. *Theriogenology*, 25(1): 150-162.

Das, S.K., Jain, G.C., Solanki V.S. and Tripathi, V.N. 1996. Efficiency of various collection methods for oocytes retrieval in buffalo. *Theriogenology*, 46: 1403-1411.

De Loos, F.A.M., Bevers, M.M. Dieleman S.J. and Kruip, A.M. 1991. Morphology of preovulatory bovine follicles as related oocyte maturation. *Theriogenology*, 35(3): 527-535.

De Loose, F.A.M., Van Vliet, C., Van Maurik P. and Kruip, T.A.M. 1989. Morphology of immature bovine oocytes. *Gamete Res.*, 24: 197-204.

De Wit, A.A.C., Wurth Y.A. and Kruip, T.A.M. 2000. Effect of ovarian phase and follicle quality on morphology and developmental capacity of the bovine cumulus-oocyte complex. *J. Anim. Sci.*, 78: 1277-1283.

Dode, M.A.N., Rodovalho, N.C. Ueno V.G. and Alves, R.G.O. 2001. Oocyte recovering from *Bos indicus* females. *Arch. Zootec.*, 50: 415-418.

Downs, S.M., Schroeder A.C. and Epping, J. J. 1986. Serum maintains the fertilizability of mouse oocyte matured *in vitro* by preventing hardening of zona pellucida. *Gamete Res.*, 15: 115-122.

Duranthon, V. and Renard, J.P. 2001. The developmental competence of mammalian oocytes: a convenient but biologically fuzzy concept. *Theriogenology*, 55(6): 1277-1289.

El-Gaafary, M.N. and Abdel-Ghaffar, A.E. 1994. *In vitro* oocyte maturation, fertilization and cleavage in Egyptian buffaloes. *Annals of AgricSciMoshtohor*, 32(4): 1801-1810.

El-Naby, Al-H, Al-shimaa., Mahmoud, Gh. M. H. K., Ahmed, Y.F., Abouel-Roos M.E.A. and Abdel-Ghaffar, A.E. 2013. Effect of season of the year and ovarian structures on oocytes recovery rate, quality and meiotic competence in Egyptian buffaloes. *Global Veterinaria*, 10: 408-412.

Eppig, J., Wigglesowrth, J. K. and Brien, M.J.O. 1992. Comparison of embryonic development competence of mouse oocytes grown with and without serum. *Mol. Reprod. Dev.*, 32: 33-40.

Eppig, J.J. 1996. Co-ordination of nuclear and cytoplasmic oocyte maturation in eutherian mammals. *Reprod Fertil Dev.*, 8: 485-489.

Ferreira, E.M., Vireque, A.A. Adona, P.R. Meirelles, F.V. Ferriani R.A. and Navarro, P.A. 2009. Cytoplasmic maturation of bovine oocytes: structural and biochemical modifications and acquisition of developmental competence. *Theriogenology*, 71: 836-848.

Fuhrer, F., Mayr, B., Schellander, K., Kalat M. and Schleger, W. 1989. Maturation competence and chromatin behaviour in growing and fully grown cattle oocytes. *J. Vet. Med.*, 36: 285-291.

Fukui, Y. and Ono, H. 1989. Effects of sera, hormones and granulosa cells added to culture medium for *in vitro* maturation, fertilization, cleavage and development of bovine oocytes. *J. Report. Fertil.* 86: 501-506.

Fulka, Jr. J., First N.L. and Moor, R.M. 1998. Nuclear and cytoplasmic determinants involved in the regulation of mammalian oocyte maturation. *Mol Hum Reprod*, 4(1): 41-49.

Funahashi, H. 1998. Cytoplasmic maturation of porcine oocytes for successful male pronuclear formation and early embryonic development. Scientific reports of the faculty of agriculture Okayama University, 87: 205-214.

Gasparrini, B., Attanasio, L. Ade Rosa, A. Monaco, E. Di Palo R. and Campanile. G. 2007. Cryopreservation of *in vitro* matured buffalo (*Bubalus bubalis*) oocytes by minimum volumes vitrification methods. *Anim. Reprod. Sci.*, 98: 335-342.

Gordon, I. 2003. Laboratory production of cattle embryos: Maturing the oocyte, 2nd edition, cambridge, MA 02138, CABI Publishing.

Gordon, I., 1990. *In vitro* maturation (IVM) and fertilization (IVF) of cattle ova. *Embryo Transfer Newsletter*, 2: 6-11.

Grondahl, C. 2008. Oocyte maturation. *Danish Medical Bulletin*, 55(1): 1-16.

Gupta, P.S.P., Ravindra, J.P. Girishkumar, V. Raghu H.M. and Nandi, S. 2005. Stimulation of *in vitro* oocyte maturation with a novel peptide isolated from follicular fluid of the buffalo (Bubalus bubalis). *Small Rumin. Res.*, 59: 33-40.

Hegab, A.O., Montasser, A.E., Hammam, A.M., Abu El-Naga, E.M.A. and Zaabel, S.M. 2009. Improving *in vitro* maturation and cleavage rates of buffalo oocytes. *Anim. Reprod.*, 6(2): 416-421.

Hunt, P.A. and Hassold, T.J. 2002. Sex matters in meiosis. Science Washington 296: 2181-2183.

Hussein, T.S., Thompson J.G. and Gilchrist, R.G. 2006. Oocyte-secreted factors enhance oocyte developmental competence. *Dev. Biol.,* 296: 514-521.

Hyttel, P., Fair, T. Callesen H. and Greve, T. 1997. Oocyte growth, capacitation and final maturation in cattle. *Theriogenology,* 47(1): 23-32.

Hyttel, P., Xu, K.P. Smith S. and Greve, T. 1986. Ultrastructure of in-vitro oocyte maturation in cattle. *J. Reprod. Fertil,* 78: 615-625.

Kadoom, A. Kh. A., 1995. *Studies on: in vitro maturation, fertilization and development of buffalo oocytes.* Ph.D. Thesis (Gynecology, Obstetrics and A.I. Faculty of Vet. Med. Alex. University.

Katska, L. 1984. Comparison of two methods for recovery of ovarian oocytes from slaughter cattle. *Anim Reprod Sci.,* 7: 461-463.

Kharche, S.D., Sharma, G.T. and Majumdar, A.C. 2005. *In vitro* maturation and fertilization of goat oocytes vitrified at germinal vesicle stage. Small Rumin. Res., 57: 81-84.

Knobil, E. and Neill, J.D. 1988. *The Physiology of reproduction.* Vol. 1, Raven Press, New York, pp: 69-102.

Krisher, R.L., 2004. The effect of oocyte quality on development. *J. Anim. Sci.,* 84: 14-23.

Kruip, T.A.M., Cran, D.G., van Beneden T.H. and Dieleman, S.J. 1983. Structural changes in bovine oocytes during final maturation in vivo. *Gamete Res.,* 8: 29-47.

Kubelka, M., Motlik, J., Fulka, J.J., Prochazka, R., Rimkevikova, Z. and Fulka, J.1988. Time sequence of germinal vesicle breakdown in pig oocytes after cycloheximide and p-amino benzamidine block. *Gamete Res.,* 19: 423-431.

Kumar, A., Solanki, V.S., Jindal, S.K., Tripathi V.N. and Jain, G.G. 1997. Oocyte retrieval and histological studies of follicular population in buffalo ovaries. *Anim. Reprod. Sci.,* 47: 189-195.

Lechniak, D., D. Kaczmarek, D. Stanislawski and Adamowicz,T. 2002. The ploidy of *in vitro* matured bovine oocytes is related to the diameter. *Theriogenology,* 57: 1303-1308.

Leibfried, L. and First, N.L. 1979. Characterization of bovine follicular oocytes and their ability to mature *in vitro. J. Anim. Sci.,* 48(1): 76-86.

Leibfried-Rutledge, M., Crister, E.S., Parrish J.J. and First, N.L. 1989. *In vitro* maturation and fertilization of bovine oocytes. *Theriogenology,* 31: 61-74.

Levesque, J.T. and Sirard, M.A. 1995. Effects of different kinases and phosphatases on nuclear and cytoplasmic maturation of bovine oocytes. *Mol. Reprod Dev.,* 42: 114-121.

Lonergan, P., Carolan C. and Mermillod, P. 1994. Development of bovine embryos *in vitro* following oocyte maturation under defined conditions. *Reprod. Nutr. Dev.*, 34: 329-339.

Marteil, G., Richard-Parpaillon L. and Kubiak, J.Z. 2009. Role of oocyte quality in meiotic maturation and embryonic development. *Reprod Biol.*, 9(3): 203-224.

Martino, A., Palomo, M.J., Mogas T. and Paramio, M.T. 1994. Influence of the collection technique of prepubertal goat oocytes on *in vitro* maturation and fertilization. *Theriogenology*, 42: 859-873.

Mayes, M. (2002). The meiotic arrest of bovine oocytes. PhD thesis, Faculty of Graduate Studies, Laval University, pp. 4-68.

Mermillod, P., Locatelli, Y., Dalbies-Tran, R., Uzbekova, S., Baril, G., Guignot, F. Perreau, C., Poulin, N., Touze, J.L., Pennetier, S., Schmaltz B. and Cognie, Y. 2006. *In vitro* production of ruminant embryos: results, limits and perspectives. Symposium COA/INRA scientific cooperation in agriculture, Tainan (Taiwan, R.O.C.). pp. 59-78.

Moor, R.M. and Trounson, A.D. 1977. Hormonal and follicular factors affecting maturation of sheep oocytes *in vitro* and their subsequent developmental capacity. *J. Reprod Fertil*, 49: 101-109.

Motlagh, M.K., Shahneh, A.Z., Daliri, M., Kohram, H. and Gharagozlou, F. 2008. *In vitro* maturation of sheep oocytes in different concen-trations of mare serum. *African J. Biotechnol.*, 7(18): 3380-3382.

Motlik, J. and Fulka, J. 1981. *In vitro* maturation of mammalian oocytes. *Ontogenez*, 12(5): 435-442.

Nandi, S., Chauhan M.S. and Palta, P. 2001. Effect of environmental temperature on quality and developmetal competence *in vitro* of buffalo oocytes. *Vet. Record.*, 148: 278-279.

Nandi, S., Ravindranatha, B.M., Gupta P.S.P. and Sharma, P.V. 2002. Timing in sequential changes in cumulus cells and first polar body extrusion during *in vitro* maturation of buffalo oocytes. *Theriogenology*, 57: 1151-1159.

Pawshe, C.H., Palanisamy, A., Taneja, M., Jain S.K. and Totey, S.M. 1996. Comparison of various maturation treatments on *in vitro* maturation of goat oocytes and their early embryonic development and cell numbers. *Theriogenology*, 46: 971-982.

Rao, B.S., Naidu, K.S., Amarnath, D., Vagdevi, R., Roa, A.S., Brahmaiah, K.V. and Roa, V.H. 2002. *In Vitro* maturation of sheep oocytes in different media during breeding and non-breeding seasons. Small Rumin. Res., 43: 1-36.

Roy, A., Razada, B.C. Tiwari, R.B.I. Andey, M.D.P. Yadavand P.O. and Sengupta, B.P. 1968. Effect of management on fertility of buffalo cows bred during summer. *Indian J. Vet. Sci.*, 38: 554-560.

Sagirkaya, H. M. Yagmur, Z. N. and Soylu, M.K. 2004. Replacement of fetal calf serum with synthetic serum substitute in the *in vitro* maturation medium: effects on maturation, fertilization and subsequent development of cattle oocytes *in vitro*. *Turk J Vet Anim Sci.*, **28**: 779-784.

Schroeder, A., Schultz, R.M., Kopf, G.S., Taylor, E.R., Becker, R.B and Eppig, J.J. 1990. Fetuin inhibit zona pellucida hardening and conversion of ZP2=ZP2f during spontaneous mouse oocyte maturation in the absence of serum. *Biol. Reprod.*, 43: 891.

Schroeder, A.C. and Eppig, J.J. 1984. The developmental capacity of mouse oocytes that matured spontaneously *in vitro* is normal. *Dev. Biol.*, 102: 493-497.

Shamsuddin, M., Larsson B. and Rodriguez-Martinez, H. 1993. Maturation-related changes in bovine oocytes under different culture conditions. *Anim Reprod Sci.*, 31: 49-60.

Shirazi, A. and Sadeghi, N. 2007. The effect of ovine oocyte diameter on nuclear maturation. *Small Rumin. Res.*, 69: 103-107.

Singh, R. and Majumdar, A.C. 1992. Chronological changes of buffalo follicular oocyte maturation *in vitro*. *Indian J. Anim. Sci.*, 82: 205-209.

Sirard, M.A., Richard, F., Blondin P. and Robert, C. 2006. Contribution of the oocyte to embryo quality. *Theriogenology*, 65(1): 126-136.

Smiljakovae, T. and Tomek, W. 2006. Meiotic maturation and *in vitro* maturation of Bovine oocytes. *Biotechnology in Animal Husbandry*, 22(1-2): 29-34.

Szollosi, D., Calarco P. and Donahue, R. 1972. The nuclear envelope: its breakdown and fate in mammalian oogonia and oocytes. *Anat. Rec.*, 174: 325-340.

Thompson, J.G., 2000. *in vitro* culture and embryo metabolism of cattle and sheep embryos. A decade of achievement. *Anim. Reprod. Sci.*, 30: 273-280.

Tomek, W., Torner H. and Kanitz, W. 2002. Comparative analysis of protein synthesis, transcription and polyadenilation of mRNA during maturation of bovine oocytes *in vitro*. *Reprod Domest Anim*, 37: 86-91.

Totey, S.M., Pawshe C.H. and Singh, G.P. 1993. *In vitro* mutation and fertilization of buffalo oocytes (*Bubalus bubalis*): Effect of media, hormones and sera. *Theriogenology*, 39: 1153-1171.

Tsafriri, A., Cao, X., Ashkenazi, H., Mottola, S., Popliker M. and Pomerantz, S.H. 2005. Resumption of oocyte meiosis in mammals: On models, meiosis activating sterols, steroids and EGF like factors. *Mol. Cell. Endocrinol.*, 234(1-2): 37-45.

Van Soom, A., Tanghe, S., De Pauw I., Maes D. and DeKruif, A. 2002. Function of the cumulus oophorus before and during mammalian fertilization. *Reprod Domest Anim*, 37(3): 144-151.

Varisanga, M.D., Sumantri, C. Murakami, M. Fahrudin D. and Suzuki, T. 1998. Morphological classification of the ovaries in relation to the subsequent oocyte quality for IVF-produced bovine embryos. *Theriogenology*, 50: 1015-1023.

Wang, Z.G., Xu Z.R. and Yu, S.D. 2007. Effects of oocyte collection techniques and maturation media on *in vitro* maturation and subsequent embryo development in Boer goat. *Czech J. Anim Sci.*, 52(1): 21-25.

Watson, A.J. 2007. Oocyte cytoplasmic maturation: A key mediator of oocyte and embryo developmental competence. *J. Anim. Sci.*, 85(E. Suppl.): E1-E3.

Wurth, Y.A., Boni, R. Hulshof S.C.J. and Kruip, T.A.M. 1992. Bovine embryo production *in vitro* after selection of ovaries, follicles and oocytes. *12th Inter. Cong. Anim. Prod.*The Hague, the Netherlands. 1: 387-389.

Yadav, B.R., Katiyar, P.K. Chauhan M.S. and Madan, M.L. 1997.Chromosome configuration during *in vitro* maturation of goat, sheep and buffalo oocytes. *Theriogenology*. 47: 943-951.

Yang, X., Kubota, C., Suzuki, H., Taneja, M., Bols P. E. and Presicce, G. A. 1998. Control of oocyte maturation in cows: Biological factors. *Theriogenology*, 49: 471-482.

Yousaf, M.R. and Chohan, K.R. 2003. Nuclear morphology, diameter and meiotic competence of buffalo oocytes relative to follicle size. *Reprod. Fertil. and Dev.*, 15(4): 223-Leibfried, M.L. and First, N.L. 1979. Characterization of bovine follicular oocytes and their ability to mature *in vitro*. *J. Anim. Sci.*, 48(1): 76-86.

Zeron, Y., Ocheretny, A. Kedar, O. Borochov, A. Sklan D. and Arav, A. 2001. Seasonal changes in bovine fertility: Relation to developmental competence of oocytes, membrane properties and fatty acid composition of follicles. *Reprod.* 121: 447-454.

Zoheir, K.M.A., Abdoon, A.S., Mahrous, K.F., Amer, M.A., Zaher, M.M., Li-Guo Y. and El-Nahass, E.M. 2007. Effects of season on the quality and *in vitro* maturation rate of Egyptian buffalo (*Bubalus bubalis*) oocytes. *J. Cell and Anim. Biol.*, 1(2): 029-033.

❑❑❑

Chapter 9

Sexing of The Sperm : An Update

SANJAY AGARWAL

Division of Veterinary Gynaecology & Obstetrics,
F.V.Sc. & A.H., S.K.U.A.S.T-J, R. S. Pura-181102, Jammu

Introduction

Reproductive biotechnologies are a set of methods, procedures or operations whose main purpose is to maximize genetic potential and to obtain more offspring, under optimal conditions, beyond the limits characteristic for the species. Among the latest-generation biotechnologies which have brought a considerable contribution to the field of reproduction are a number of assisted reproductive technologies (ART), such as: in vitro fertilization (IVF), intravaginal culture of oocytes (INVO), intracytoplasmic sperm injection (ICSI), transgenesis, embryo sexing, and sperm sexing technology (Faber *et al.*, 2003; Vintila, 2005).

Today, there are relatively easy and rapid procedures to determine the sex-chromosomal composition of individual sperm (e.g. fluorescence in situ hybridization with a DNA probe; Fugger, 1999) or the sex ratio of a population of sperm. The quickest, easiest (with the right equipment), and most reliable of these is analysis of the proportions of X- and Y-sperm as determined by DNA content using flow cytometry (Pinkel *et al.*, 1982; Garner *et al.*, 1983; Welch and Johnson, 1999), the precision of which often is under-appreciated due to its statistical nature.

Management schemes for live stock production can benefit from sex preselection because of the ability to plan matings for a specific sex. Making the sex determination prior to conception is the most cost-effective means of achieving the desired result. The only accurate and potentially cost effective approach for achieving sex preselection at the present time involves separating the X- from the Y-chromosome-bearing sperm followed by its use for artificial insemination (AI) or for in vitro fertilization (IVF) with subsequent embryo transfer (ET).

In addition to more rapid genetic progress from the use of sexed sperm or embryos there are additional advantages of management and facility flexibility. As with the utilization of most assisted reproductive practices (IVF–ET), sexed sperm for production of livestock of preselected sex is dependent on efficiency, economics, effectiveness, and ease of use. Widespread use of sexed sperm will increase, as each of these factors is considered and the technology is developed to such an extent as to become available on demand. At the present time economics and ease of use remain goals to be attained.

History of Sperm Sexing

The preselection of the sex of offspring prior to conception has aroused great interest since ancient times. The first attempts to control and determine the sex of the offspring were described by certain philosophers of ancient Greece. Democritus of Abdera (approx. 460-360 BC) believed that male offspring originated in the right testicle and female offspring in the left testicle (Garner and Seidel, 2008). Moreover, it was believed that male fetuses developed more frequently in the right uterine horn, while the female fetuses – in the left uterine horn. According to this assumption, in the case of both the human and animal species, in order to obtain offspring of the desired sex, one of the testicles was removed (Taton *et al.*, 1970). The first description of semen or "*sperma*" was made by Hippocrates from Kos (c.460-c.377 BC) (Taton *et al.*, 1970), who claimed that "*sperma*" plays a key role in the development of the product of conception. Strong "*sperma*" produces male descendants, while weak "*sperma*" - female descendants. However, all these hypotheses were based on an empirical tradition, without any scientific research basis to certify their validity (Windsor *et al.*, 1993). Even though Anton van Leeuwenhoek, in 1677, described the spermatozoon for the first time using a simple microscope. In the first half of the 20th century advances in the biological sciences, especially genetics, resulted in numerous discoveries, including identification of the sex chromosomes. Michael Frederick Guyer, in 1910, gave the first accounts regarding the microscopic identification of sex chromosomes in mammals, the actual scientific approaches referring to preselection of the sex of offspring prior to conception were undertaken only in the twentieth century (Seidel, 2012). Lush (1925) conducted one of the first significant attempts to pre-select sex with semen of pigs and rabbits. But his study, based on centrifugation, failed to attain any significant skewing of the sex ratio. With the advance of time many new theories and methods were developed for the efficient sexing of semen. More than a dozen approaches to sexing sperm have been attempted, but convincing results were not produced. First attempts to separate X and Y bearing sperms were made by Gledhill *et al.* (1976) through analytical flow cytometry. The major breakthrough was development of flow cytometry/cell sorting in the early 1980s Collaboration between Oklahoma State University (OSU) and Lawrence Livermore National Laboratory (LLNL) demonstrated the potential use of flow cytometry to convincingly identify X- and Y-sperm populations based on their DNA content differences. Highly condensed sperm nucleus with unusual shape of sperm head caused difficulty in quantitative fluorescence measurement and thus marginal successful in separation of sperms. Pinkel *et al.* (1982) overcome sperm heads associated problems through development of flow cytometry precisely for sperm sorting that orient the sperm heads with flattened side. Sperm sorting technology was first developed at Lawrence Livermore National Laboratory, where Pinkel *et al.* (1982) separated the X and O sperm nuclei of the *Microtus oregoni*, which have 9% DNA content difference of its sex determining chromosomes. In 1989, the USDA Beltsville Research Center group reported production of live offspring from sex-sorted, living rabbit sperm. In 1989, a major breakthrough in sperm sexing was reported by Johnson *et al.* (1989) through production of live offspring from sex sorted live rabbit spermatozoa after surgical insemination in the oviduct. Application to domestic livestock sperm separation was then implemented at Beltsville Agriculture Research Centre, USDA. Flow cytometry for sperm sexing is a patent procedure and patency lies with the M/s X–Y–INC Colorado (USA). Through license of sexing technology to many companies, sexed semen has been produced for nearly 18 different breeds of cattle in USA and in European countries.

Current State of The Art

Although sperm are substantially identical phenotypically, one method of sexing sperm at about 90% accuracy is available, namely flow cytometry/cell sorting after staining sperm with the fluorescing DNA-binding dye, Hoechst 33342 (Johnson and Welch, 1999). This technique exploits the difference in DNA content of X- and Y-chromosome-bearing sperm, which is in the order of 3–5%, depending on the species. Heroic efforts at optimizing flow cytometry/cell sorting (Johnson and Welch, 1999) plus optimizing conditions of artificial insemination (AI) have enabled AI of heifers with sexed sperm resulting in about 90% accuracy of sex of resulting offspring, but in some cases at reduced fertility (Seidel *et al.*, 1999). This procedure is commercialized for many species, initially for applications, such as in vitro fertilization (IVF) and manufacture of valuable transgenic animals.

Flow-Cytometric Sorting of Semen

Sexing of X- and Y-chromosome bearing sperm based on the difference in DNA content is the most reliable and repeatable method to produce sex-preselected animals. Since the first report by Johnson *et al.* (1989) in rabbits, flowcytometric sexing technology has been shown to be efficacious in several species including buffalo (Johnson, 2000; Seidel and Garner, 2002; Maxwell *et al.*, 2004; Lu *et al.*, 2007; Liang *et al.*, 2008). The earlier studies failed to notice difference in the DNA content between X- and Y- bearing sperm because of random orientation of the sperm in the flow-cytometer fluid stream (Johnson and Welch, 1999). The first flow sorting of sperm for purpose of isolating X from Y-bearing spermatozoa was reported by Pinkel *et al.* (1982). The work was done by using a specially built orienting flow cytometer using sperm from the creeping vole (*Microtus oregoni*). The difference in DNA content between X and Y sperm of many animals has been quantified (Johnson, 2000; Parrilla *et al.*, 2004; O'Brien *et al.*, 2005; Lu *et al.*, 2013).

Sexing Efficiency

The efficiency of sexing achieved with the aid of the flow cytometer depends to a large extent on the parameters of the sorting system, but also on the quality of semen (Parrilla *et al.*, 2001). Consequently, only 30% of the spermatozoa in one ejaculate are subjected to sexing, while the remaining 70% are lost in the stages before, during, and after sorting (Seidel and Garner, 2002).

The deterioration degree of spermatozoa subjected to the sexing technique

The entire sorting process includes several critical stages that may affect the qualitative parameters of the spermatozoa. In addition to these stages, careful handling and preparation of semen samples before and after sorting are also essential in maintaining motility, viability, and fertilizing capacity of the sexed spermatic cells.

Therefore, during the sorting process, factors responsible for diminished quality are:

- Dilution and marking procedures with H-42 (Durand and Olive, 1982).
- UV rays (Libbur *et al.*, 1987).
- Flow pressure (Suh and Schenk, 2003).
- Electrostatic field and electric charge (Suh and Schenk, 2003).
- Potential causes like temperature, osmolality, pH, and sterility of the media and laboratory glassware (Seidel and Garner, 2002).

Potential Improvements in Flow Cytometry/Cell Sorting For Sexing Sperm

Damage caused to the sperm cell: in addition to the stress of cryopreservation, sperm are subjected to many mechanical and chemical stresses during sorting (Garner *et al.*, 2001). These includes:

- Exposure of sperm to the DNA-binding dye, Hoechst 33342.
- Exposure of sperm to electromagnetic energy from laser light and emitted fluorescence, when sperm are interrogated for DNA content.
- Inelastic shear-forces, as sperm exit the sorter nozzle at about 90 km/h.
- Stretching sperm, as the exiting stream breaks into droplets.
- Abrupt deceleration from 90 to 0 km/h, as sperm encounter the air–liquid interface of the collection tube and.
- Post-sorting processing, such as centrifugation to concentrate sperm (Schenk *et al.*, 1999).

Opportunities to improve current procedures for sexing sperm, includes:

- Development or use of different DNA-binding dyes.
- Improving the speed of cell sorting.
- Increase the concentration of sorted sperms.
- Modifying the physical characteristics of the sorting process.
- Concentrating sorted sperm without centrifugation, etc.
- Designing simpler and more robust unipurpose sperm sorters.
- Economical and easy to operate.

Other Attempts for Separation of X and Y- Bearing Spermatozoa

Albumin Gradient

Moruzzi (1979) reported that Y chromosome is smaller than X chromosome. Ericsson *et al.* (1973) though first reported the successful separation of X and Y-bearing spermatozoa using an albumin gradient, but Maxwell *et al.* (1984) observed that there was no much difference in the ratio of X- Y- bearing spermatozoa.

Centrifugal Counter Current Distribution based on Density Characteristics

Meistrich (1982) reported that the difference in density between X-bearing bovine spermatozoa and Y-bearing bovine spermatozoa to be only 0.0007 g/cm^3. Ollero *et al.* (2000) tried to sex ram spermatozoa by centrifugal counter current distribution.

Counter Current Galvanic Separation

The selection can be done by the application of a suitable micro-ampere current that will attract Y-bearing spermatozoa to the anode and X-bearing spermatozoa to the cathode (Bhattacharya, 1977). Foote (1985) used the same technique but could not succeed in producing any significant alteration of sex ratio.

Free Flow Electrophoresis

It is based on the hypothesis that the electric charge on the surface of X-bearing spermatozoa differs from that of Y-bearing spermatozoa, uses an electric field to separate spermatozoa into the two major classes (Kaneko *et al.*, 1984). Inseminations with semen separated by this technique yielded disappointing results. Blottener *et al.* (1983) found a birth rate of 50.4% female calves in inseminations carried out on 1185 animals using semen enriched in X-bearing spermatozoa. Another drawback of this technique was an associated reduction in motility of the sperm after being subjected to electrophoresis.

Genetic Approaches

Seidel (1988) suggested a genetic approach for sperm sexing. Herrmann *et al.* (1999) demonstrated this concept by placing part of this genetic system on the Y chromosome using transgenic procedures.

Hormonal Manipulation for Sexing of Spermatozoa

Barat and Leger (1979) and James (1980) reported that administration of clomiphene citrate and or/ gonadotrophins resulted in 8.7% lowering of sex ratio.

Immunological Sexing of Semen

Blecher *et al.* (1999) carried out a study in this aspect. Immunization of male and female rabbits by injecting sperm preparations with Freund's incomplete adjuvant subcutaneously was done to raise antibodies to sperm membrane proteins. The anti-sperm antisera obtained from the female rabbit were putative "anti-Y" and those obtained from male rabbit were "anti-X" antisera. Sperm doses after suitable treatment were mixed with either of these antisera and incubated for 60 min at 38.5ºC and 5% CO_2. It was found that only the "anti-X" antisera resulted in agglutination of spermatozoa whereas the "anti-Y" antisera failed to show any agglutinations in the spermatozoa. The agglutinated sperm population was separated from the free-swimming sperm by glass wool filtration and the free-swimming sperm population (potentially Y-bearing spermatozoa) was isolated. Bovine embryos were produced *in vitro* using the isolated sperm population and blastocysts were sexed cytogenetically. The results indicated that 92% of the sexed embryos were male thus marking the technique as one of the potential methods of sperm sorting. This method has to be validated by further experiments and another constraint is that the method was successful in isolating Y-bearing spermatozoa only and attempts to isolate X-bearing spermatozoa by agglutinating Y-bearing spermatozoa was not successful. Beerli *et al.* (2008) reported that each cellular protein can be recognizable by a set of antibodies, so an immunological approach may be more efficient for detecting proteins with a low concentration. Yang *et al.* (2014) confirmed that the putative XSSAb contained SSAbs that captured three candidate SSP spots. This provides a potentially more efficient method for sorting sperm and lays a foundation for future search for SSPs. However, additional studies are needed to further confirm the specificity of XSSAb and identify candidate proteins of SSPs.

Percoll Density Gradient

In this method, semen is allowed to penetrate a percoll column. Iwasaki (1988) reported that the technique was not effective in separation of X or Y-bearing spermatozoa.

Separation on the Basis of Presence of HY Antigen

Attempts to inactivate the Y sperm by immunological methods have been tried on the H-Y antigen (Goldberg *et al.*, 1971). Zavos (1985) reports the usefulness of H-Y antigen in selecting only the X-bearing rabbit spermatozoa. Hoppe and Koo (1984) suggested that X- and Y-bearing spermatozoa probably share the same surface antigen. Watchel (1983) demonstrated the presence of HY antigen in the membrane of both X and Y spermatozoa under normal circumstances, which was confirmed by Hendrikssen *et al.* (1993) hence, sexing the spermatozoa on the basis of HY antigen is not effective.

Sperm Sorting based on Volumetric Differences

Van Munster *et al.* (1999) used interference microscopy and subsequent image analysis to demonstrate a difference in sperm head volume that matched differences in DNA content between X and Y-bearing bovine spermatozoa. Unfortunately, the potential purity of spermatozoa separated using volumetric measurements cannot exceed 80% purity of either sex based on theoretical considerations.

Swimming Patterns under Laminar Flow

Sarkar *et al.* (1984) reported that Y-bearing spermatozoa swim differently and more quickly than X-bearing spermatozoa in a column of flowing media. The feasibility of this technique is questionable as only 10 % of the total number of spermatozoa placed in the system could be recovered.

Applications of sexing sperm

1. ***Human Medicine and Gender Balancing of Families :*** Preventing sex chromosome specific genetic diseases and gender balancing within families are the predominant anticipated applications of sexing human sperm. In Romania they have generated a high interest in both human and veterinary medicine. Currently, there are over 10.000 known diseases that are genetically determined or conditioned and which affect the human population, of which 370 are sex-linked. Haemophilia, Duchenne and Becker muscular dystrophies, G6PD deficiency, the Lesch-Nyhan syndrome, and agammaglobulinemia are just some of the most serious diseases caused by different genes located on the X chromosome and which generally occur only in male children. Thus, in order to

avoid such situations, in the case of families with a history of sex-linked diseases, the preselection of the child's sex prior to conception would be the only viable solution (Cuevas *et al.*, 2002).

2. ***Production Agriculture*** : In cattle farms, where in the case of dairy breeds the farmers prefer female offspring (Xu, 2014) as compared to beef breeds, where male offspring are preferred Thus, at an approximately equal rate of male and female new-borns, as in the case of artificial insemination with non-sexed semen, half the offspring belong to an unwanted sex category, raising and then selling the cattle in question to slaughter houses being basically unprofitable. Thus, the spread of artificial insemination with sexed semen brings about great advantages for both farm categories (Xu, 2014).
3. ***Biotechnological Application*** : It includes production of animals to clone and transgenic applications. In the latter case, huge costs are incurred with each animal, and sex of founder animals as well as subsequent individuals in transgenic breeding schemes usually will be worth specifying.
4. ***Sport Animals*** : The use of sexed semen also raises a great interest in the case of animals destined for elite sports, such as horses, dogs, elk and even camels, as well as animals used for hunting. In both cases, male offspring are preferred (Seidel, 2003). A related non-sport application is to produce antler velvet for medicinal and nutritional purposes and herbal remedies.
5. ***Zoo Animals*** : Such applications include optimizing breeding schemes of zoo animals to prevent inbreeding and rescuing endangered species.
6. ***Research*** : In many areas of research, predetermination of sex would reduce costs, partly by decreasing the number of animals required. Research on sexing sperm also can produce important basic information in other areas, such as immunology (e.g. Blecher *et al.*, 1999). Another example is that the need to optimize use of limited number of sexed sperm has driven research to improve in vitro storage of sperm, procedures to cryopreserve sperm, and methods of insemination (Schenk *et al.*, 1999; Seidel *et al.*, 1999).
7. ***Genetic Improvement*** : The acceleration of reproduction management and the improvement of genetic level can be improved by this technology for livestock population.

Limitations of Sperm Sexing

- Expensive method
- Time consuming
- Potential harmful effects on spermatozoa
- Considerable damage to sperm
- Not able to sex semen with 100% purity
- Reduced fertility

Introducing sexed sperm to the bovine AI industry

- Sexed sperm should increase efficiency of producing meat and milk, create new opportunities for AI to take market share away from natural breeding, and improve the welfare of cattle.
- There are two possible broad objectives in introducing sexed sperm for bovine AI: profit and satisfying the needs/wants of the owners of cattle.
- Another market for sexed bovine sperm is special applications such as IVF and insemination of superovulated donors.

Concern before commercializing sexed sperm for species other than cattle

- The value of end product per year from a dairy cow is at least 20× that of a sheep, but costs to sex sperm of each species are similar.
- Basic physiology also differs among species. It is not unusual to obtain 1000 doses of semen for AI per week from a bull, whereas 1000 doses per year might be more realistic for stallions or boars.
- Cryopreservation of bovine semen is routinely successful for the vast majority of bulls; cryopreservation is much less successful for nearly every other species, partly due to huge male to male differences.
- Infrastructure for delivering semen to the end producer is well-developed for cattle in many countries, and hardly developed at all for most other species in most countries.

Ethical Issues and Legislation

The mammalian sex selection does not involve any distinctive ethical concerns, but condition is different in case of humans. Sex selection in humans, can be separated into two distinct reasons: medical and non-medical. If sex selection for medical reasons is carried out in order to avoid the transmission of X-linked genetic diseases to the next generation, sex selection for non-medical reasons is done mostly in order to satisfy parental desires. Sex selection for medical reasons is accepted as ethical in many countries but for non-medical reason has been subjected to intense debate in many countries (Strange, 2010). Moreover, article 14 of the Convention on Human Rights and Biomedicine of 1997 states that "the use of techniques of medically assisted procreation shall not be allowed for the purpose of choosing a future child's sex, except where serious hereditary sex-related disease is to be avoided" (Dondorp *et al.*, 2013). Parental freedom of choice is the most common and strongest argument in favour of non-medical sex selection. While, the primary arguments against allowing preconception sex selection for non-medical reasons are that can lead to sex-ratio imbalance and distortions in birth order, is inherently sexist and violates human dignity, misuse the medical resources for nonmedical purposes, and can induce risks of perpetuation of social injustice and discrimination. Also, many critics who argue against non-medical sex selection believe that the possibility to preselect the sex of a child prior to conception is akin to "playing God" by interfering with the natural process of reproduction and what is "natural" ought to be appreciated as part of divine creation. Furthermore the position of the Roman Catholic Church is that the ability to give birth to children is the expression of marital love and should not be isolated from the sexual act (Kalfoglou *et al.*, 2013; Liao, 2005).

Conclusion

Sexed sperm produced by current methods may remain an imperfect product for some years. Currently, the main imperfections can include lowered fertility, high cost, and only 90% accuracy for practical purposes. As the magnitude of these imperfections is reduced, commercialization will increase, first in niches, where one sex is worth considerably more than the other, and then, more widely.

References

Amann, R.P. (1999). Issues affecting commercialization of sexed sperm. *Theriogenol.*, **52:** 1441–1457.

Barat, J. and Leger, D. (1979). Avenir des grossesses obtenuse après stimulation de I' ovultion. A propos de 519 grossesses. *J. Gynecol. Obslel. Biol. Reprod.*, **5:** 332.

Bhattacharya, B. C., Shome, P., Gunther, A. H. and Evans, B. M. (1977). Successful separation of X and Y spermatozoa in human and bull semen. *Int. J. Fert.*, **22:** 30-35.

Blecher, S. R., Howie, R., Li, S., Detmar, J. and Blahut, L. M. (1999). A new approach to immunological sexing of sperm. *Theriogenol.*, **52:** 1309-1321.

Blottener, S., Nehring, H., Jenichem, W. and Peter, W. (1983). Use of carrier free deflection electrophoresis in experiments for separation of sperm genotypes. *Arch. Exp. Veterinamed.*, **37:** 641-655.

Cuevas, I., Llacer, J., Ten, J., Mendiola, J. and Bernabeu, R (2002). Current situation of sex selection. *Situación actual de la selección de sexo.*, **19(5):** 337.

Dondorp, W., DeWert, G., Pennings, G., Shenfield, F., Devroey, P., Tarlatzis, B., Barri, P. and Diedrich, K. (2013). Task Force on Ethics and Law 20: Sex selection for non-medical reasons. *Hum Reprod.*, **28(6):** 1448-1454.

Doyle, S.P. (2000). Determination of the impacts and effectiveness of sexed semen utilization in commercial beef cattle production. Ph.D. Thesis. Colorado State University, Fort Collins, CO.

Durand, R. E. and Olive, P. L. (1982). Cytotoxicity, mutagenicity and DNA damage by Hoechst 33342. *J. Histochem. Cytochem.*, **30(2)** : 111-116.

Faber, D. C., Molina, J. A., Ohlrichs, J. A., Vander Zwaag, D. F. and Ferre, L.B. (2003). Commercialization of animal biotechnology. *Theriogenol.*, **59(1):** 125-38.

Foote, R. H. (1985). Normal development of fetuses resulting from Holstein semen processed for sex separation. *Theriogenol.*, **24:** 197-202.

Fugger, E. (1999). Clinical experience with flow cytometric separation of human X- and Y-chromosome bearing sperm. *Theriogenol.*, **52:** 1435–1440.

Garner, D. L., Gledhill, B. L., Pinkel, D., Lake, S., Stephenson, D., Van Dilla, M. A. and Johnson, L. A. (1983). Quantification of the X- and Y-chromosome-bearing sperm of domestic animals by flow cytometry. *Biol. Reprod.*, **28:** 312–321.

Garner, D. L., Schenk, J. L. and Seidel Jr., G. E. (2001). Chromatin stability in sex-sorted sperm. In: Andrology in the 21st Century, Proceedings of the VIIth International Congress of Andrology, Montreal, Canada, Short Communications, pp. 3–7.

Garner, D.L. and Seidel, Jr. G. E. (2008). History of commercializing sexed semen for cattle. *Theriogenol.*, **69(7):** 886-895.

Goldberg, E. H., Boyse, E. A., Bennet, D., Scheid, M. and Carswell, E. A. (1971). Serological demonstration of H-Y (male) antigen on mouse sperm. *Nature*, **232:** 478-480.

Hendriksen, P. J. M., Tieman, M., Van der Lende, T. and Johnson, L. A. (1993). Binding of anti H-Y monoclonal antibodies to separated X and Y chromosome bearing porcine spermatozoa. *Mol. Reprod. Dev.*, **35:** 189-96.

Hermann, B. G., Koschroz, B., Wertz, K., McLaughlin, K. J. and Kispert, A. (1999). A protein kinase encoded by the *t complex responder* gene causes non-mendalian inheritance. *Nature*, **402:** 141-146.

Hoppe, P. C. and Koo, G. C. (1984). Reacting mouse sperm with monoclonal H-Y antibodies does not influence sex ratio of eggs fertilized *in vitro*. *J. Reprod. Immunol.*, **6:** 1-9.

Iwasaki, S., Shioya, I., Masuda, H., Hanada, A. and Akahara, T. (1988). Sex ratio of early embryo fertilized *in vitro* with spermatozoa separated by percoll. *Theriogenol.*, **30:** 1191-1198.

James, W. (1980). Gonadotrophins and the human secondary sex ratio. *Br. Med. J.*, **281**: 711.

Johnson, L. A. (2000). Sexing mammalian sperm for production of offspring: the state of- the-art. *Anim. Reprod. Sci.*, **61:** 93–107.

Johnson, L. A. and Welch, G. R. (1999). Sex preselection: high-speed flow cytometric sorting of X- and Y- sperm for maximum efficiency. *Theriogenol.*, **52:** 1323–1341.

Johnson, L. A., Flook, J. P. and Hawk, H. W. (1989). Sex preselection in rabbits: live births from X- and Y- sperm separated by DNA and cell sorting. *Biol. Reprod.*, **41:** 199–203.

Kalfoglou, A. L., Kammersell, M., Philpott, S. and Dahl, E. (2013). Ethical arguments for and against sperm sorting for non-267 medical sex selection: a review. *Reprod. Biomed.*, **26:** 231-239.

Kaneko, S., Oshiro, S., Kobayashi, T., Itzuka, R. and Mohri, H. (1984). Human X- and Y- bearing sperm differ in cell surface sialic acid content. *Biochem. Biophys. Res. Commun.*, **124:** 950- 955.

Liang, X. W., Lu, Y. Q., Chen, M. T., Zhang, X. F., Lu, S. S., Zhang, M., Pang, C. Y., Huang, F. X. and Lu, K. H. (2008). *In vitro* embryo production in buffalo (*Bubalus bubalis*) using sexed sperm and oocytes from ovum pick up. *Theriogenol.*, **69:** 822–826.

Liao, S. M. (2005). The ethics of using genetic engineering for sex selection. *Med. Ethics*, **31:** 116–118.

Libbus, B. L., Perreault, S. D., Johnson, L. A. and Pinkel, D. (1987). Incidence of chromosome aberration in mammalian sperm stained with Hoechst 33342 and UV-laser irradiated during flow sorting. *Mutat. Res.*, **182(5):** 265.

Lu, Y. Q., Liang, X. W., Zhang, M., Wang, W. L., Kitiyanant, Y., Lu, S. S., Meng, B. and Lu, K. H. (2007). Birth of twins after *in vitro* fertilization with flow-cytometric sorted buffalo *(Bubalus bubalis)* sperm. *Anim. Reprod. Sci.*, **100:** 192–196.

Lu, Y., Lu, S. S., Zhang, M. and Xiaogan, Y. (2013). Sperm sexing in buffalo using flow cytometry. *Buffalo Bull.*, **32:** 22-30.

Lush, J. L. (1925). The possibility of sex control by artificial insemination with centrifuged spermatozoa. *J. Agri. Res.*, **30:** 893-913.

Maxwell, W. M. C., Evans, G., Hollinshead, F. K., Bathgate, R., De Graaf, S. P., Eriksson, B. M., Gillan, L., Morton, K. M. and O'Brien, J. K. (2004). Integration of sperm sexing technology into the ART toolbox. *Anim. Reprod. Sci.*, **83:** 79–95.

Maxwell, W. M. C., Meddoa, G. and Shite, I. G. (1984). Post thawing survival of motile ram sperm after isolation by layering on protein columns. *Theriogenol.*, **21:** 601-606.

Meistrich, M. (1982). Potentials and limitations of physical methods for separations of sperm bearing an X or Y chromosome prospects for sexing Mammalian sperm. Colorado Associated Univ. Press, Boulder, Colorado. pp. 145-163.

Moruzzi, J. F. (1979). Selecting a mammalian species for the separation of X- and Y-chromosome bearing spermatozoa. *J. Reprod. Fert.*, **57:** 319-323.

O'Brien, J. K., Stojanov, T., Heffernan, S. J., Hollinshead, F. K., Vogelnest, L., Maxwell, W. M. C. and Evans, G. (2005). Flow cytometric sorting of non-human primate sperm nuclei. *Theriogenol.*, **63(1):** 246–259.

Ollero, M., Perez-Pe, R., Gargallo, I., Morlanes, S., Osada, J., Muino-Blanco, T. and Cebrian-Perez, J. (2000). Separation of ram spermatozoa bearing X and Y chromosome by centrifugal countercurrent distribution in an aqueous two phase system. *J. Androl.*, **21:** 921-928.

Parrilla, I. Vazquez, J. M. Centurion, F., Roca, J., Gil, M. A. and Lucas, X. (2001) Effect of high-speed flow sorting on sperm motility pattern of boar sperm. *Theriogenol.*, **55:** 501.

Parrilla, I., Vazquez, J. M., Roca, J. and Martinez, E. A. (2004). Flow cytometry identification of X- and Y-chromosome bearing goat sperm. *Reprod. Dom. Anim.*, **39:** 58–60.

Pinkel, D., Gledhill, B. L., Lake, S., Stephenson, D. and Ven Dilla, M. A. (1982). Sex preselection in mammals? Separation of sperm bearing Y and 'O' chromosome in the vole *Microtus Oregoni. Sci.*, **218:** 904-906.

Pinkel, D., Lake, S., Gledhill, G.L., Van Dilla, M.A., Stephenson, D. and Watchmaker, G. (1982). High resolution DNA content measurements of mammalian sperm. *Cytometry*, **3:** 1–9.

Sarkar, S., Jolly, D. J., Friedman, T. and Jones, O. W. (1984). Swimming behaviour of X and Y human sperm. *Differentiation*, **27:** 120-125.

Schenk, J. L., Suh, T. K., Cran, D. G. and Seidel Jr., G. E. (1999). Cryopreservation of flow-sorted bovine spermatozoa. *Theriogenol.*, **52:** 1375–1391.

Seidel Jr., G. E. (2003). Economics of selecting for sex: the most important genetic trait. *Theriogenol.*, **59:** 585–598.

Seidel Jr., G. E., Schenk, J. L., Herickhoff, L. A., Doyle, S. P., Brink, Z., Green, R. D. and Cran, D. G. (1999). Insemination of heifers with sexed sperm. *Theriogenol.*, **52:** 1407–1420.

Seidel, G. E. Jr. (1988). Sexing spermatozoa and embryos – state of the art. In: Proceedings of XI international congress of animal reproduction and artificial insemination (Dublin) Vol. **5**, University College, Dublin. pp. 136-144.

Seidel, G. E. JR. (2003). Sexing mammalian sperm: intertwining of commerce, technology, and biology. *Anim. Reprod. Sci.*, **79 (3-4):** 145-146.

Seidel, G. E. Jr. (2012). Sexing Mammalian Sperm – Where Do We Go from Here? *J. Reprod. Dev.*, **58(5):** 505-509.

Seidel, G. E. Jr. and Garner, D. L. (2002). Current status of sexing mammalian spermatozoa. *Reprod.*, **124(6):**733-743.

Seidel, G. E. Jr., Schenk, J. L., Herickoff, L. A., Doyle, S. P., Brink, Z., Green, R. D. and Cran, D.G. (1999). Insemination of heifers with sexed sperm. *Theriogenol.*, **52:** 1407–1420.

Strange, H. (2010). Non-medical sex selection: ethical issues. *Br. Med. Bull.*, **94:** 7–20.

Suh, T. K. and Schenk, J. L. (2003). Pressure during flow sorting of bull sperm affects post-thaw motility characteristics. *Theriogenol.*, **59:** 516.

Taton, R., Armaldez Rbeaujeu, J., Beaujouan, G., Bloch, R., and Bourgey, L. (1970). Stiinta antica si medievala – de la origini la 1450. Vol.I, Ed. Stiintifica Bucuresti, **212-214**; 205-214.

Van Munster, E. B., Stap, J., Hoebe, R. A., Te Meerman, G. J. and Aten, J. A. (1999). Difference in sperm head volume as a theoretical basis for sorting X- and Y-bearing spermatozoa: potentials and limitations. *Theriogenol.*, **52**: 1281-1293.

Vintila, I. (2005). Transferul de embrioni °i biotehnologii asociate. *Ed. Orizonturi Universitare Timisoara*, 11.

Watchel, S. S. (1983). Sex specific transplantation antigens in species other than mouse. In: HY antigen and the biology of sex determination, Gruene and Stratton, New York. pp. 22-37.

Welch, G. R. and Johnson, L. A. (1999). Sex preselection: laboratory validation of the sperm sex ratio of flow sorted Xand Y-sperm by sort reanalysis for DNA. *Theriogenol.*, **52:** 1343–1352.

Windsor, D. P., Evans, G. and White, I. G. (1993). Sex predetermination by separation of X and Y chromosome-bearing sperm: A review. *Reprod. Fertil. Dev.*, **5(2):** 155-171.

Xu, Z. Z. (2014). Application of liquid semen technology improves conception rate of sex-sorted semen in lactating dairy cows. *J. of Dairy Sci.*, **97(11):** 7298–7304.

Yang, W. C., Sang, L., Xiao, Y., Zhang, H. L., Tang, K. Q. and Yang, L. G. (2014).Tentative identification of sex-specific antibodies and their application for screening bovine sperm proteins for sex-specificity. *Mol. Biol. Rep.*, **41(1):** 217-23.

Zavos, P. (1985). Sperm separation attempts via the use of albumin gradients in rabbits. *Theriogenol.*, **23:** 875.

□□□

Chapter 10

Pig As a Large Animal Model for Study on Drug Metabolism and Regulation

ARUN KUMAR DE[1*], A. KUNDU[2], JAI SUNDER[1], M.S.KUNDU[1] D. BHATTACHARYA, PERUMAL, P., T. SUJATHA AND LAWRENCE B SCHOOK[3,4]

[1] Animal Science Division ICAR-Central Island Agricultural Research Institute, Port Blair, Andaman and Nicobar Islands; [2] Director, ICAR-Central Island Agricultural research Institute, Port Blair, Andaman and Nicobar Islands; [3] Department of Animal Sciences, University of Illinois at Urbana-Champaign, Urbana, Illinois, USA; [4] University of Illinois Cancer Center, Urbana, Illinois, USA; * **Correspondence:** biotech.cari@gmail.com

Introduction

Predicting the fate of a drug in a particular patient and his or her subsequent response is still a vision and far away from application in routine clinical practice. Recognizing the sources and understanding the factors that contribute to the extraordinary pharmacokinetic and pharmacodynamic variability within and between individuals remains a challenge of particular importance for drugs with narrow therapeutic index. Drug metabolizing enzymes (DMEs) play central roles in the metabolism, elimination, and detoxification of xenobiotic introduced into the body. Analysis of the pig genome has revealed high homology between porcine and human genes, including genes associated with drug metabolism (Schook *et al.,* 2015). The characterization of porcine drug metabolism genes and the genes involved in regulating drug metabolism can provide insights into human drug metabolic diseases and individual variability of responses toward a drug.

Major reasons that contribute to the failure of a drug in preclinical and clinical studies are toxicity and efficacy. The adverse effects of new drugs are often not discovered until preclinical animal safety studies or even clinical trials; 40% of drugs drop out in preclinical animal studies and 89% of those that reach clinical trials fail (McKim,

2010). There is a critical need for more predictive and reliable *in vitro* testing methods. A good *in vitro* model can identify issues related to toxicity early in the discovery process thereby saving millions of dollars.

Why pig?

The pig was first used in biomedical research in ancient Greece and has quickly grown into an important biomedical research tool over the past few decades (Schook *et al.*, 2015). Pigs have genetic and physiological traits very similar to humans, which make them one of the most useful and versatile animal models. Similarity in size and physiology to humans allow pigs to be used for many experimental approaches not feasible in mice. The whole genome sequence of pig revealed that pig has similar genes involved in drug metabolism. Therefore, pig may be a very good model of drug metabolism and toxicity assessment.

Drug Metabolizing Enzymes

Drug metabolizing enzymes (DMEs) play central roles in the metabolism, elimination, and detoxification of xenobiotics introduced into the body. Analysis of the pig genome has revealed high homology between porcine and human genes, including genes associated with drug metabolism. The characterization of porcine drug metabolism genes and the genes involved in regulating drug metabolism can provide insights into human drug metabolic diseases and individual variability of responses toward a drug. Most of the tissues and organs express diverse and various DMEs, including phase I and phase II metabolizing enzymes and phase III transporters. These DMEs can be present in abundance at the basal level, or expression can be induced after exposure to drugs (Xu *et al.*, 2005).

Phase I metabolism includes oxidation, reduction, hydrolysis, and hydration. Enzymes catalyzing these reactions are found in virtually all tissues, especially in the hepato-intestinal axis (Xie *et al.*, 2004). Phase I DMEs consist primarily of the cytochrome P450 (CYP) superfamily and are found abundantly in the liver, GI tract, lung, and kidney(Nelson *et al.*, 2003). In humans, five CYP gene families, CYP1, CYP2, CYP3, CYP4, and CYP7, are believed to play crucial roles in hepatic and extrahepatic metabolism and elimination of xenobiotics and drugs (Lewis, 2003). The products of phase I metabolism are generally more polar and more readily excreted than the parent compounds and are often substrates for phase II enzymes (Xie *et al.,* 2004). The pig is an appropriate animal model for the investigation of drug disposition, as the transporters and CYP enzymes are very similar to those in humans (Anzenbacher *et al.,* 1998). The CYPs constitute the major enzyme family capable of catalyzing the oxidative biotransformation of most drugs and other lipophilic xenobiotics and are of particular relevance for clinical pharmacology. Several of these CYP subfamilies have been characterized for the pig and minipig (Bode *et al.,* 2010). They include the main liver enzyme of drug metabolism (CYP3A) in comparable amounts and activity levels to humans (Anzenbacher *et al.,* 1998).In addition, the porcine pregnane X receptor protein regulates CYP3A, which metabolizes almost half of the prescription drugs in humans, and has higher homology to that of humans than the mouse gene product (Gray *et al.,* 2010). That makes the pig a better model than the mouse to determine, if a compound is toxic to humans. For these reasons, pigs are considered an ideal model for evaluating the safety of pharmaceuticals and biopharmaceuticals (Forster *et al.,* 2010).

Phase II metabolism involves conjugation with endogenous hydrophilic compounds to increase polarity and water solubility, thereby increasing excretion in the bile and urine, resulting in a detoxification effect. The phase II metabolizing or conjugating enzymes, consisting of many superfamily of enzymes including sulfotransferases (SULT) and UDP-glucuronosyl transferases (UGT), DT-diaphorase or NAD(P)H:quinone oxidoreductase (NQO) or NAD(P)H: menadione reductase (NMO), epoxide hydrolases (EPH), glutathione S-transferases (GST) and N-acetyltransferases (NAT) (Xu *et al.,* 2005). Each superfamily of phase II DMEs consists of families and subfamilies of genes encoding the various isoforms with different substrate specificity, tissue and developmental expression, as well as inducibility and inhibitory by xenobiotics. In general, conjugation with phase II DMEs generally increases hydrophilicity, and thereby enhances excretion in the bile.

Phase III transporters play crucial roles in drug absorption, distribution, and excretion. They include P-glycoprotein, multidrug resistance–associated protein, organic anion transporting polypeptide 2, and ABC transporters. They are expressed in many tissues, including liver, intestine, kidney, and brain.

In vitro Model of Drug Metabolism

Metabolism of a drug or xenobiotics is critical for its pharmacokinetic properties, and the liver is the main organ of drug or xenobiotics biotransformation (Lübberstedt et al.; Tuschl *et al.*, 2009). The cytochrome P450 (CYP) isozymes expressed in the hepatic tissue constitute the major enzyme family capable of catalyzing the oxidative biotransformation of most drugs and lipophilic xenobiotics (Brandon *et al.*, 2003). Primary human hepatocytes are considered the gold standard model for drug metabolism and toxicity studies as they provide a complete picture of the metabolic fate of xenobiotics *in vitro* (Lübberstedt *et al.*, Brandon *et al.*, 2003). However, primary human hepatocytes have limited and unpredictable availability and undergo early and variable phenotypic alterations in culture (Guillouzo *et al.*, 2007). Most of the human liver cell lines have poor or fractional CYP expression (Gómez-Lechón *et al.*, 2001). To date, the lack of a reliable animal model for assessment of drug toxicity and metabolism is a major limitation in early high throughput screening of xenobiotics. Immunological and physiological differences between rodents and humans represent major constraints for the use of rodent-based models in drug screening. Therefore, a large animal model surrogate for human hepatocytes is a very important improvement over the current methods for early screening of novel drugs and xenobiotics.

Over the years, the pig has gained increasing importance as a biomedical model due to similarities in size, anatomy and physiology with humans (Schook *et al.*, 2015). CYP enzymes have been extensively studied in pigs and enzymes equivalent to human P450 (eg. CYP1A, 2A6, 2E1, 3A4) have been identified in pig liver (Soucek *et al.*, 2001; Szotáková *et al.*, 2004; Achour *et al.*, 2011). The sequence homology between human and porcine P450 enzymes is striking, ranging from 72 to 95 % (Achour *et al.*, 2011). Biotransformation data indicate that the CYP1A, 2A and 3A enzyme systems seem to be functionally very similar between pigs and humans (Bogaards *et al.*, 2000; Nebbia *et al.*, 2003).

Conclusion

Pigs are increasingly being used as the major non-rodent animal species of choice in biomedical research, especially in preclinical toxicological testing of pharmaceuticals. The popularity of pig, especially minipig in pharmacology, pharmacokinetic, and toxicological safety evaluation experiments has increased very rapidly over recent years. The pig is a true omnivore like human and because of this, the physiology of digestion and metabolic processes in the liver are also similar to humans. Pig can be used as a laboratory model for human xenobiotic metabolism without the requirement to induce biotransformation enzymes.

References

Achour, B., Barber, J., and Rostami-Hodjegan, A. (2011). Cytochrome P450 Pig Liver Pie: Determination of Individual Cytochrome P450 Isoform Contents in Microsomes from Two Pig Livers Using Liquid Chromatography in Conjunction with Mass Spectrometry. Drug Metab. Dispos. 39: 2130–2134.

Anzenbacher P, Soucek P, Anzenbacherova E, Gut I, Hruby K, Svoboda Z, et al. Presence and Activity of Cytochrome P450 Isoforms in Minipig Liver Microsomes. Comparison with Human Liver Samples. Drug Metab Dispos. 1998; 26: 56–59.

Bode G, Clausing P, Gervais F, Loegsted J, Luft J, Nogues V, et al. The utility of the minipig as an animal model in regulatory toxicology. J Pharmacol Toxicol Methods. 2010; 62: 196–220.

Bogaards, J.J., Bertrand, M., Jackson, P., Oudshoorn, M.J., Weaver, R.J., Bladeren, P.J. van, et al. (2000). Determining the best animal model for human cytochrome P450 activities: a comparison of mouse, rat, rabbit, dog, micropig, monkey and man. Xenobiotica. 30: 1131–52.

Brandon, E.F.A., Raap, C.D., Meijerman, I., Beijnen, J.H., and Schellens, J.H.M. (2003). An update on in vitro test methods in human hepatic drug biotransformation research: pros and cons. Toxicol. Appl. Pharmacol. 189: 233–46.

Forster R, Ancian P, Fredholm M, Simianer H, Whitelaw B, Project SG of the R. The minipig as a platform for new technologies in toxicology. J Pharmacol Toxicol Methods. 2010; 62: 227–35.

Gómez-Lechón, M.J., Donato, T., Jover, R., Rodriguez, C., Ponsoda, X., Glaise, D., et al. (2001). Expression and induction of a large set of drug-metabolizing enzymes by the highly differentiated human hepatoma cell line BC2. Eur. J. Biochem. 268: 1448–59.

Gray MA, Pollock CB, Schook LB, Squires EJ. Characterization of porcine pregnane X receptor, farnesoid X receptor and their splice variants. Exp Biol Med (Maywood). 2010;235: 718–36. doi:10.1258/ebm.2010.009339.

Guillouzo, A., Corlu, A., Aninat, C., Glaise, D., Morel, F., and Guguen-Guillouzo, C. (2007). The human hepatoma HepaRG cells: a highly differentiated model for studies of liver metabolism and toxicity of xenobiotics. Chem. Biol. Interact. 168: 66–73.

Lewis DF V. Human cytochromes P450 associated with the phase 1 metabolism of drugs and other xenobiotics: a compilation of substrates and inhibitors of the CYP1, CYP2 and CYP3 families. Curr Med Chem. 2003; 10: 1955–72.

Lübberstedt M, Müller-Vieira U, Mayer M, Biemel KM, Knöspel F, Knobeloch D, et al. HepaRG human hepatic cell line utility as a surrogate for primary human hepatocytes in drug metabolism assessment in vitro. J Pharmacol Toxicol Methods. 63: 59–68.

McKim JM. Building a tiered approach to in vitro predictive toxicity screening: a focus on assays with in vivo relevance. Comb Chem High Throughput Screen. 2010; 13: 188–206.

Nebbia, C., Dacasto, M., Rossetto Giaccherino, A., Giuliano Albo, A., and Carletti, M. (2003). Comparative expression of liver cytochrome P450-dependent monooxygenases in the horse and in other agricultural and laboratory species. Vet. J. 165: 53–64.

Nelson DR, Zeldin DC, Hoffman SMG, Maltais LJ, Wain HM, Nebert DW. Comparison of cytochrome P450 (CYP) genes from the mouse and human genomes, including nomenclature recommendations for genes, pseudogenes and alternative-splice variants. 2003; 450: 1–18.

Schook LB, Collares T V, Darfour-Oduro KA, De AK, Rund LA, Schachtschneider KM, et al. Unraveling the swine genome: implications for human health. Annu Rev Anim Biosci. Annual Reviews; 2015;3: 219–44. doi:10.1146/annurev-animal-022114-110815.

Soucek, P., Zuber, R., Anzenbacherová, E., Anzenbacher, P., and Guengerich, F.P. (2001). BMC Pharmacology. 450: 2–6.

Szotáková, B., Baliharová, V., Lamka, J., Nozinová, E., Wsól, V., Velík, J., et al. (2004). Comparison of in vitro activities of biotransformation enzymes in pig, cattle, goat and sheep. Res. Vet. Sci. 76: 43–51.

Tuschl G, Hrach J, Walter Y, Hewitt PG, Mueller SO. Serum-free collagen sandwich cultures of adult rat hepatocytes maintain liver-like properties long term: a valuable model for in vitro toxicity and drug-drug interaction studies. Chem Biol Interact. 2009; 181: 124–37.

Xie W, Uppal H, Saini SPS, Mu Y, Little JM, Radominska-Pandya A, et al. Orphan nuclear receptor-mediated xenobiotic regulation in drug metabolism. Drug Discov Today. 2004;9: 442–9. doi:10.1016/S1359-6446(04)03061-2.

Xu C, Li CY-T, Kong A-NT. Induction of phase I, II and III drug metabolism/transport by xenobiotics. Arch Pharm Res. 2005;28: 249–68. Available: http://www.ncbi.nlm.nih.gov/pubmed/15832810.

□□□

Chapter 11

Molecular and Bioinformatics Perspective for *Pasteurella multocida* Infection (Haemorrhagic Septicaemia) and Pasteurellosis in Animals

HARSHIT VERMA[1], MAYANK RAWAT[2] AND RISHENDRA VERMA[3]

[1] Assistant Professor, Department of Veterinary Microbiology, College of Veterinary and Animal Sciences, Meerut- (UP); [2] Principal Scientist, Division of Standardization; [3] ICAR-Emeritus Scientist, ICAR-Indian Veterinary Research Institute, Izatnagar-243 122 (UP), E-mail: rishendra_verma@yahoo.com

Historically, *Pasteurella multocida*, was first described during 1887-89 when Rivolta and Rivolee reported outbreak in fowl and it was followed by report of a disease in Cattle by Bollinger in Germany and its causative bacterium was isolated by Kit in 1885, along with other reports like septicaemia in rabbits (Gaffky, 1881), swine plague (Loeffler, 1886). The name *Pasteurella* was suggested by Trevisan in 1887 after Louis Pasteur who elucidated etiology of fowl cholera. Since 1889, the research on *P. multocida* has been undertaken by various laboratories in South East Asia and India both for academic research and by investigators of ICAR- All India, Network Programme (AINP) started in the year 2000 involving Centres at Anand, Chennai, Guwhati, Izatnagar, Ludhiana, Palampur and Thrissur. The major thrust of research on *P. multocida* has been development of a vaccine against haemorrhagic septicaemia and pasteurellosis in animals in India. The occurrence of *P. multocida* and its significance in animals in India depended on either outbreaks of pasteurellosis or on the basis of post-mortem of animals. Haemorrhagic septicaemia (HS) form of Pasteurellosis in buffalo and cattle is caused by specific *P. multocida* serotype 6:B (B:2) in Asia and serotype 6:E (E:2) in Africa. The Asian serotype B:2 causes acute classical HS in cattle and buffaloes characterized by oedamtous swelling of the head and neck, and swollen haemorrhagic lymph nodes (Carter and De Alwis, 1989).

HS has been considered to be one of the most economically important diseases of South East Asia (Bain, 1963). Recently, simultaneous occurrence of foot-and-mouth disease (FMD) and haemorrhagic septicaemia (HS) has been recorded for last 3-4 years, which are economically devastating diseases in India. This was manifested in Moga district of Punjab in 1998 where large numbers of animals died. It was believed that FMDV produced a transient immunosuppression that predisposed the animals to *P. multocida* infection resulting into the death of the animal. These authors contended combined vaccination with FMD + HS (Chhabra *et al.*, 2004).

P. multocida

According to the description byWilson and Ho (2013)in his review, *P.multocida* is a member of the family *Pasteurellaceae,* which comprises the genera, *Pasteurella, Haemophilus,* and *Actinobacillus,* and three recently proposed additions *Mannheimia, Gallibacterium* and *Lonepinella. Pasteurellaceae* have already been renamed: *Histophilussomni* (formerly *Haemophilus somnus, H. agni,* and *H.ovis*), *Mannheimia* (formerly *Pasteurella*) *haemolytica, Bibersteinia* (formerly *Pasteurella*) *trehalosi, Actinobacillus* (formerly *Haemophilus*) *pleuropneumoniae, Actinobacillus* (formerly *Pasteurella*) *ureae, Aggregatibacter* (formerly *Actinobacillus*) *actinomycetemcomitans, Aggregatibacter aphrophilus* (formerly *Haemophilus aphrophilus* and *H. paraphrophilus*), *Aggregatibacter* (formerly *Haemophilus*) *segnis, Avibacterium* (formerly *Haemophilus*) *paragallinarum, Avibacterium* (formerly *Pasteurella*) *gallinarum, Avibacterium* (formerly *Pasteurella*) *volantium, Avibacterium* (formerly *Pasteurella*) *avium, Basfia* (formerly *Mannheimia*) *succiniciproducens,* and *Gallibacterium* (formerly *Pasteurella*) *anatis.*

P. multocida is a small, gram-negative, nonmotile, non–spore-forming coccobacillus with bipolar staining features. The bacteria typically appear as single bacilli on Gram stain; sometimes as pairs and short chains. There are five serogroups of *P. multocida* based on capsule antigens as "A", "B", "D", "E" and "F" and further classified into 16 serotypes based primarily on LPS antigens using the Heddleston scheme (Carter, 1955; Heddleston *et al.*,1972), The new capsule of serogroup of *P. multocida* serogroup F, isolated from Turkeys in different areas of United States was reported (Rimler and Rhoades, 1987).

Prevalence of Serotypes of *P. multocida* in Animal and Avian species

The prevalence of *P. multocida* in different animal and avian species in India during November 2000 and July 2003 was reported in which out of 418 samples, 206 bacterial cultures were identified as *P. multocida. P.multocida* were identified on the basis of cultural, morphological and biochemical characteristics. 206 cultures of *P. multocida* were isolated from animals e.g. cattle, buffalo, sheep, goat, pig and rabbit, wild animals e.g. leopard and deer and avian species including chicken, duck, quail, turkey, goose. Serotyping of *P. multocida* isolates showed presence of various serotypes (A:1, A:3, A:1,3, B:2, D:1) and the study revealed varied serotypes among livestock (Kumar *et al.*, 2004). It has been reported that both, serotypes A:1 and A:3 were associated with fatal pneumonia and septicemia of cattle and buffaloes in India. Multilocus sequence typing (MLST), a sequence-based typing method for bacterial pathogens, is currently the best method for long-term epidemiological study and to understand the population structure of the bacteria. This investigation was carried out to study the diversity of *Pasteurella multocida* isolates circulating in India. Ten different sequence types (ST) identified in this study are ST 122 from cattle, goat, mithun and pig; ST 50 from pig; ST 9 from cattle and sheep; ST 229 from cattle and goat; ST 71 and ST 277 from cattle; and ST 129, ST 280, ST 281 and ST 282 from avian species. Of these, ST 277, ST 280, ST 281 and ST 282 were identified for the first time. The analysis of results provides novel epidemiological information on the circulation of multiple STs across India. The majority of STs or their variants identified in this study have already been reported from different parts of the globe. This suggests that probably transboundary spread of strains across countries and continents has occurred across evolutionary time and is still happening. The isolation of ST 122 from small ruminants and pigs suggests that these species may be included in the preventive vaccination policy for effective control of haemorrhagic septicaemia in India (Sarangi *et al.*, 2014).

Molecular variability in *P. multocida* isolates

Out of five isolates from outbreak of HS affecting buffaloes in India, repetitive extragenic palindromic (REP)-PCR, enterobacterial repetitive intergenic consensus (ERIC-)-PCR and single- primer PCR differentiated all five isolates into different profiles. It was important observation of the authors that all five isolates involved in outbreak were found to have a genetic profile different from standard *P. multocida* (P_{52}) (Biswas *et al.*, 2004). Three out of five had similar profiles while two had a different profile. This study reported involvement of multiple strains of *P.multocida* in a single outbreak of *P. multocida.* A PCR assay targeting the *hyaC-hya*D gene identified fifty isolates belonging to serogroup-A showed identical RFLP analysis of PCR products after digestion with *Bg/*II (Gautam *et al.*, 2004). In Vietnam, *P. multocida* isolates from concurrent outbreaks of HS in cattle, buffaloes and pigs were found identical (ACIAR; Project IDAS2/1995/006). *P. multocida* (serotype B:2) isolates (35) from different animals were found similar phenotypically and genotypically, when subjected to differentiation by restriction endonuclease (REA), ribotyping and randomly amplified polymorphic-DNA (RAPD)-PCR analysis (Dutta *et al.*, 2004). Sixty seven (67) field isolates of *P. multocida* originated from different animals species and geographical regions of India examined by repetitive extragenic palindromic sequence based PCR (REP-PCR) yielded 23 profiles, which were clustered into eight groups. There was no host-specific, type-specific, region-specific or pathogenicity-specific pattern. The REP profiles of isolates from wild animals were similar to profiles from domestic animals. Two common bands were present in all the isolates irrespective of somatic or antigenic types (Saxena *et al.*, 2006).

Whole Genome Sequence (WGS) of *P. multocida*

May *et al.*, (2001) explored genetic content of virulence genes in *P. multocida* and reported the first complete genome sequence of the avian strain Pm70. The Pm70 strain was isolated in 1970 from the oviduct of a chicken in Texas. This strain belongs to serotype F:3 and not A:3 as reported earlier and is not virulent in chickens. Therefore, they sought to sequence the genomes of two virulent strains, namely *P. multocida* strains X73 (serotype A:1) and P1059 (serotype A:3). Both strains are highly virulent in turkeys, chickens, and other poultry species. A recent study by Moustafa *et al.*, (2015) using genome sequences of 11 HS strains and four other *P. multocida* strains revealed 96 HS-specific genes which could promote the development of disease-specific diagnostic tests. The genome sequence of *Pasteurella multocida* subsp. *gallicida* strain Anand1_poultry was achieved by a shotgun sequencing strategy using 454 pyrosequencing. The sequences were assembled with the Newbler assembler (454 Life Sciences). The GS reference mapper was used to create contigs (with *Pasteurella multocida*

Pm70 used as a reference genome, and the resulting contigs were subjected to the NCBI Prokaryotic Genome Annotation Pipeline (http://www.ncbi.nlm.nih.gov/genomes/static/Pipeline.html). The data generated from the genomic library contained 96,816 reads, and the assembly generated a 2,017,480-bp-long single chromosome with a G+C content of 40.23% (Ahir *et al.*, 2011).

Whole-genome shotgun sequencing of *P. multocida* HN06, a toxigenic serogroup D strain isolated from a diseased pig in China was performed by using the Illumina Solexa platform. A total of 4,792,617 paired-end reads were generated from a genomic DNA library with 300 - to 500-bp fragments, giving an ~ 360-fold coverage of the genome. All reads were *de novo* assembled using the Velvet package, and 61 contigs of more than 500 bp were generated. Gaps between contigs were closed by primer walking. Protein-coding sequences (CDSs) were predicted by use of the programs Glimmer and GeneMarks. tRNAs and rRNAs were identified using tRNAscan-SE and RNAmmer, respectively. *P. multocida* HN06 consists of a circular chromosome with 2,402,218 bp and a plasmid, pHN06, with 5,360 bp.The average GC contents of the chromosome and plasmid are 40.2% and 47.5%, respectively (Lieu *et al.*, 2012).

The genome sequencing of *P. multocida* strains P1059 and X73 was achieved via 454 pyrosequencing of a shotgun library. The sequences were assembled *de novo* with Newbler V2.6 (454 Life Sciences), and Pm70 was used as a reference strain for scaffolding; the resulting assembly generated 2.30 Mbp (40.21% GC, 24 contigs, 18 contigs> 500 bp, N_{50} 256,544) and 2.26 Mbp (40.30% GC, 39 contigs, 28 contigs >500 bp, N_{50} 137,372) genomes for P1059 and X73, respectively (Abrahante *et al.*, 2013). The strains 2213 and 3213 of *P. multocida* were isolated from the blood of carcasses of two buffaloes (*Bubalis bubalis*) that died during outbreaks of HS disease from two different farms in South Karnataka, India. Both isolates belonged to capsular serogroup B as determined by using the multiplex capsular PCR system. Genomic DNAs of both strains were isolated in India using the Qiagen DNA extraction kits. Whole-genome sequencing was per-formed using the IlluminaMiSeq platform. RAST annotation of strain 2213 using strain 36950 as a reference produced a full genome of 2,309,333 bp carrying 2,163 coding sequences classified into 425 metabolic or virulence subsystems and 59 predicted RNAs. Strain 3213 produced a genome or 2,307,438 bp carrying 2,160 coding sequences that were classified into 424 subsystems and 57 predicted RNAs (Abhrante *et al.*, 2014).

This is the first whole-genome sequence of *Pasteurella multocida* isolate from north India. Strain VTCCBAA264, a B:2 serotype, was isolated from the morbid intestinal content of a buffalo (*Bubalus bubalis*) calf, which died of high fever and respiratory distress on an organized buffalo dairy farm. The genome sequencing was achieved by 454 pyrosequencing of a shotgun library. The sequence was assembled *de novo* using Newbler V2.6. A total of 123,415 reads were generated using the GS FLX Titanium system, giving ~23 × coverage of the genome. The data generated 78 contigs ranging in size from 710 to 319,560 bp, with a total size of 2,280,332 bp, an N_{50} of 65,447 bp, and a Q40 of 99.65%. Annotation was carried out against strain Pm70 using the RAST serve (Vaid *et al.*, 2014).

Comparative genome analysis of 33 *P. multocida* strains revealed the pangenome compositions of *P. multocida*. Phylogeny of *P. multocida* was closely associated with serotyping rather than other factors like host origin or geographical location. A comprehensive analysis was done to investigate genetic content and diversification of virulence-associated genes in *P. multocida*. Their findings indicated that evolutionary dynamics of pathogenic *P. multocida* were driven by positive Darwinian selection and homologous recombination. Their study provided valuable targets for future researches on the mechanism of adaptive evolution and the host-pathogen interaction in *P. multocida* (Cao *et al.*, 2017).

Pathogenesis/Virulence

Pasteurella species are among the most prevalent commensal and opportunistic pathogens found worldwide in domestic and wild animals Pasteurellosis (symptomatic infection with *Pasteurella*) is a high-impact disease in livestock, according to the World Organisation for Animal Health (OIE) (www.oie.int). *P. multocida* organisms reside in the nasopharynx of cattle and buffalo as a commensal and whenever there is immunosuppression in the host, it causes HS. *P. multocida* pathogenesis has been reviewed by Harper *et al.* (2006). According to Harper *et al.* (2006), the key virulence factors identified to date include capsule and lipopolysaccharide. The capsule is responsible for bacterial avoidance of phagocytosis and resistance to complement, while LPS is critical for bacterial survival in the host. A number of other virulence factors have been identified by both directed and random mutagenesis, including *P. multocida* toxin, putative surface adhesions and iron acquisition proteins (Harper *et al.*, 2006).

In an experiment, after intranasal infection of eight buffaloes with a culture of a field isolate of *P. multocida* serotype B:2, three animals succumbed to the disease at 26-30h post infection (p.i.) and five survived. Rectal temperatures of infected animals rose to a peak at about 10h p.i. and surviving animals showed a second peak in rectal temperature at 36 p.i. Endotoxin was present only in serum of non-surviving animals 3-5h before death or killing during which time concentrations rapidly increased, correlating with the development of overt clinical signs and reductions in rectal temperature, concentrations of white blood cells, serum thyroxine, iron, copper and zinc an increase in serum haptaglobin and cortisol and the detection of a low-grade bacteraemia. A strong acute phase response was maintained in surviving animals with a progressive rise in serum haptaglobin over 96p.i, a slow rise in serum copper concentration from 24h p.i. and an increase, from about 65 p.i., in serum alpha1-acid glycoprotein. The findings demonstrated that a progressive endotoxaemia and associated sequelae correlated with the development of over HS disease and sudden death of buffalo (Horadagoda *et al.*, 2001). The authors contended a major contribution of terminal endotoxaemia to the outcome of disease and indicated that future control strategies should aim at preventing the onset of endotoxaemia. This may involve the use of specific anatagonists against endotoxin, related cytokines and other humoral mediators, such have been applied to other endotoxin-mediated diseases in animals and man (Olson *et al.*, 1995).

P. multocida appears to be one of the most complex and fascinating organism. The pathogenesis of the disease is a result of complex interactions between host factors, (e.g. species, age, immune status) and specific virulence factors which includes LPS, capsule, adhesions, outer membrane (Boycee and Alder, 2000). Mice are used to study pathogenesis of HS using mortality, mean death time and bacterial multiplication in vital organs after infection with live *P. multocida*. It has been found that ten bacteria are enough to cause mortality in mice and the organism multiplies rapidly in respiratory epithelium and disseminated to other vital organs *viz* liver and spleen suggesting the important role of mouse model in investigating the pathogenesis and challenge studies during vaccine development (Khrab and Charan, 2013).

The study was undertaken to examine the blood cytokine expression profiles (TNF-α, IL-1β, and IL-6), bacterial colonization and histopathological changes of intraperitoneally and subcutaneously challenged vaccinated and unvaccinated mice with 10^2 CFU of *P. multocida* P_{52}. The observations were made at 6, 12, 18, 24 h and 48 h intervals. Real-time PCR based blood cytokine profiles (TNF-α, IL-1β, and IL-6) measurement revealed a significantly higher amount of pro-inflammatory cytokines expression in the unvaccinated challenged group of mice than the vaccinated challenged group. There was heavy bacterial load in all organs of mice *viz.* trachea, lung, spleen, within 6 h of challenge in both vaccinated and unvaccinated group of mice, but bacterial load increased in the unvaccinated challenged group of mice with respect to time, whereas the load were constant in the vaccinated challenged group. Histopathological changes were mild in the vaccinated challenged group of mice in comparison to the unvaccinated challenged group. There was no significant difference in the bacterial load, histopathological changes and cytokines expression when challenged through different routes (Singh *et al.*, 2017).

The cell-invasive capacity of *P. multocida* B:2 may be a virulence property related to its ability to translocate from the respiratory tract into the blood stream (Othman *et al.*, 2012). *P. multocida* isolates possess type IV fimbriae (pili) as one of the major virulence factors based on their role in adhesion to host surfaces and subsequent pathogenesis. The gene of Indian *P. multocida* isolates (n=8) originated from different animal (buffalo, sheep, goat, pig) and avian host species (chicken, turkey, duck, quail) were amplified, cloned, sequenced and compared with available fimbrial protein sequences in GenBank/ publications (n=22) to understand its variability with respect to geography/host/serogroup/disease specific patterns. Multiple sequence alignment revealed highly conserved N-terminus α-1 helix region and heterogeneous C-terminus (68–137 aa) comprised of β-strand regions (β1, β2, β3, β4) with conserved two pairs of cysteine residues. Interestingly, an existence of absolute homogeneity among the *P. multocida* isolates that caused haemorrhagic septicaemia in bovines and septicaemic pasteurellosis in sheep and goats was noticed. Pig isolates had 99.3 % homogeneity. On contrary, more diversity (35.8%) was observed among isolates that caused fowl cholera in avians irrespective of identical capsular/somatic serogroup and similar host species. Phylogenetic analysis based on nucleotide sequences of < i > ptfA</i> gene revealed formation of mixed clusters with isolates representing different disease conditions as well as serogroups irrespective of country of origin which indicated the possible role of cross-species transmission among different animal/avian species. The study indicated highly conserved and host specific fimbriae among animal species than relatively divergent fimbriae among avian species (Shivchandra *et al.*, 2013).

Various pathogenic bacterial strains belonging to the family Pasteurellaceae have several surface exposed virulence factors including VacJ/VacJ-like lipoproteins. vacJ gene encoding for VacJ outer membrane lipoprotein of different *P. multocida* strains (n = 10) were amplified, sequenced and compared with available VacJ/VacJ-like sequences (n=45) of Pasteurellaceae members. Comparative multiple sequence analysis at amino acid level indicated absolute homogeneity of VacJ lipoprotein among different *P. multocida* strains. However, heterogeneity (18.0– 89.9%) of VacJ lipoprotein was noticed among members of Pasteurellaceae. A predicted lipobox motif (L-3-[A/S/T/V]-2-[G/A]-1-C) was found to be conserved between 12-32aa residues at N-terminus among all VacJ sequences. Bioinformatic analysis indicated that VacJ was a chromosomal gene product exposed on the bacterial surface, possibly essential for either physiological or pathogenicity process of Pasteurellae and distributed widely among *P. multocida* serogroups. The study indicated potential possibilities of using absolutely conserved VacJ lipoprotein either as 'signature gene/protein' in developing diagnostic assay or as a recombinant subunit vaccine for *P. multocida* infections in livestock (Shivachandra, 2014). Identification of outer membrane proteins (OMPs) is important to understand the bacteria structure and function, host-pathogen interaction, development of novel vaccine candidates, and diagnostic antigens. The key antigens of *P. multocida* B:2 isolate causing haemorrhagic septicaemia (HS) in animals are not clearly defined. P_{52} strain of *P. multocida* serotype B:2 was grown *in vitro* under iron-rich and iron-limited condition. The OMPs were extracted by sarkosyl method followed by SDS-PAGE and the proteins were identified by MALDI-TOF/MS analysis. In total, 22 proteins were identified, of which 7 were observed exclusively under iron-limited condition. Most of the high molecular weight proteins (TbpA, HgbA, HgbB, HasR, IroA, and HemR) identified in this study were involved in iron acquisition. Some hypothetical proteins (HP-KCU-10206, HP and AAUPMB 08244, HP AAUPMB 21592, HP AAUPMB 19766, AAUPMB 11295) were observed for the first time in this study which could be unique to serotype B:2. Further functional *in vivo* study of the proteins identified may be explored for their utility in developing diagnostics and vaccine against HS (Prasanna vadhana *et al.*, 2014).

Mice were infected with *P. multocida* (1.6 x 103 cfu, intrapeitoneal) to evaluate host gene expression profile at early and late stages of infection using high throughout microarray transcriptome analyses. Several differentially expressed genes (DEGs) at both the time points were identified in *P. multocida* infected spleen, liver and lungs. Functional annotation of these DEGs showed enrichment of key pathways, such as TLR, NR-kB, MAPK, TNF, JAKSTAT and NOD like receptor signaling pathways. Several DEGs overlapped across different KEGG pathways indicating a crosstalk between them. The predicted protein – protein interaction among these DEGs suggested, that the recognition of *P. multocida* LPS or outer membrane comonents by TLR4 and CD14, results in intracellular signaling via MyD88, IRAKs and/or TRAF6 leading to activation of NFkB and MAPK pathways and associated cytokines (Priya *et al.*, 2017).

Development of Diagnosis

The "bipolar" staining of *P. multocida* is known well which is considered relatively easy field test on the blood or impression smear. The "Gold standard" method for diagnosis is isolation of the causative agent. Therefore, *P. multocida* can be isolated in laboratory on *in vitro* employing suitable agar based media like.

The Indian *P. multocida* isolates for their antigenic typing were sent to FAO HS Reference Laboratory for South East Asia, Veterinary Research Institute, Sri Lanka. Under ICAR All India Network Project on Haemorrhagic septicaemia (AINP-HS), a capacity building has taken place to type *P. multocida* isolates by genus specific or capsule specific PM-PCR. A total of eighty three (83) isolates of *P. multocida* recovered from different animal species *viz.* cattle, buffalo, sheep, goat, rabbit, pig, duck, chicken, turkey and emu were subjected to PM-PCR. The isolates found positive in PM-PCR gave a specific band of 460 bp in agarose gel electrophoresis. The capsular typing of all isolates was done by multiplex PCR using capsular types A, B, D, E and F specific primers.The isolates, which revealed specific amplicons of 1044 bp, 760 bp, 657 bp and 851 bp were categorized into serogroups A, B, D and F, respectively. Among 83 isolates, 41 isolates belong to serotype A, 35 isolates to serotype B, 4 isolates to type D while 3 isolates belongs to type F. The isolates of Cap A type were from cattle, sheep, goat, pig, duck, poultry, turkey and emu while, type B were from cattle, buffalo, sheep, pig and rabbit. The type D was found in sheep and type F were from sheep (Annual Report, AINP-HS, 2011).

Vaccines

The contribution of Indian Veterinary Research Institute, Izatnagar in development of vaccine against HS is unparallel. Verma and Jaiswal (1998) have reviewed Haemorrhagic septicaemia vaccines. Inactivated plain bacterin, agar-wash vaccine, alum-precipitated vaccine, aluminium hydroxide gel vaccine, adjuvanted vaccine, adjuvanted *vis-à-vis* other vaccines, multiple emulsion vaccine, low volume HS vaccine, purified capsular extract vaccine and live vaccines e.g. attenuated vaccine, chemically altered live vaccine, temperature-sensitive mutant, outer membrane protein (OMP), combined vaccines, experimental idiotype vaccine, autogenous vaccine have been attempted. The development of different kinds of *P. multocida* vaccines is shown in the Table 1.

Table 1. Development of Haemorrhagic septicaemia vaccines in India

S.No.	Vaccine	Duration	Reference
1	Heat killed lyson (0.25%)	6 weeks	Baldrey, 1907
2	Heat-killed broth culture glycerine extract of old	70 % Protection immunity	Allen, 1929
3	Sensitized vaccine	4 weeks	Baldrey, 1911-12
4	Agar wash vaccine	4 months	Rau & Govil, 1950
5	a) Alum precipitated broth b) Mineral oil adjuvant broth	6 months 1 year	Iyer *et. al.*, 1955 Iyer & Rao, 1959s
6	Alum precipitated synthetic medium	Not studied	Allen, 1955
7	Purified capsular antigen vaccine	7 months 556 days	Dhanda, 1959
8	Oil adjuvant yeast extract	2 years & 4 months	Dhanda *et al.*, 1956, 1958, 1969
9	Multiple emulsion vaccine	9 months 1 year 1 year	Mittal *et al.*, 1979 Yadav & Ahuja, 1981-83 Verma & Jaiswal, 1997

Source: Verma Rishendra (1998)

The fact remains that it is the alum precipitated HS vaccine is rampantly used in India which is manufactured by State Veterinary Biological Units inspite of the fact it offers immunity of 3-4 months and thus, there is need of two times vaccination of animals in a year. M/S Indian Immunological Ltd, Hyderabad manufactured a combined HS and Black Quarter vaccine (HS +BQ).

Another development in vaccine against pasteurellosis in pigs has taken place (Harshit, 2013). *P. multocida* ("Soron") strain isolated from an outbreak of septicaemic deaths in pigs was used for development of a vaccine candidate against pig pastuerellosis. Cattle strain *P. multocida* P_{52} was used to compare the performance of vaccine made up from Soron strain. Both of these strains showed presence of h*gbB*, p*fhA*, n*anH*, p*tfA*, and *tbPA* virulence genes. SDS-PAGE analysis of cell wall of strains showed about 15 major protein bands whereas western blot analysis with 21 day Soron immunized pig serum, showed 16, 33, 47, 63 and 83kDa polypeptides in both strains. The double emulsion (W/O/W) vaccine containing 2.5 mg inactivated antigenic mass of either Soron or P_{52} strain in the internal aqueous phase studied in pigs by direct challenge showed the vaccines were protective against challenge up to 270th day. The duration of immune responses were monitored at 3, 6 and 9 months post immunization in pigs. Vaccines induced a serum ELISA IgG response that peaked on 60 DPI, which declined gradually up to 270th DPI in both vaccines. Vaccines induced a low grade cell-mediated immune response (CMI). The results in pigs showed that Soron would be a potential candidate for the vaccine against pasteurellosis and recommends use of a homolgous strain of *P. multocida* in pigs.

The vaccine is manufactured for pig pasteurellosis with cattle *P. multocida* P_{52} strain since there is no availability well characterized strain of Pig origin of *P. muloticda*. There is lack of information on atrophic rhinitis, pasteurellosis in sheep and goats in India. The alum precipitated HS vaccine is the major prophylaxis given to cattle and buffaloes.

A complete deletion of aroA in the *P. multocida* P_{52} vaccine strain, replacing the gene with a kanamycin resistance gene cassette was achieved. The developed mutant, $P_{52}\Delta$aro, was highly attenuated in mice and rabbits. The mutant failed to grow in Pasteurella minimal medium without the aromix supplement. Wild-type and mutant strain showed similar morphological and biochemical properties. In addition, mutant strain was also confirmed as *P. multocida* serotype B:2 by genus and serotype specific PCR. *In vivo* studies showed that $P_{52}\Delta$aro mutant was quickly removed from the system and no pathological lesions were observed in liver, spleen and lung. Immunization of mice and rabbits with $P_{52}\Delta$aro conferred significant level of protection. Rabbits served as a better model than mice for immunogenicity studies. (Chaudhary *et al.*, 2012).

References

1. AbrahanteJuan E., Timothy J. Johnson, Samuel S. Hunter, Samuel K. Maheswaran, Melissa J. Hauglund, Darrell O. Bayles , Fred M. Tatum, Robert E. Briggs (2013) Draft Genome Sequences of Two Virulent Serotypes of Avian *Pasteurella multocida.* Genome Announc. 1(1) : e00058-12. doi : 10.1128/genomeA.00058-12.
2. Abrahante, J.E., Veeregowda B. M., Hoglapur, S. S., Briggs, R. E. Maheswaran, S. K., and S. Sreevatsan (2014). Draft Genome Sequences of Two *Pasteurella multocida* Strains Isolated from Buffaloes in India with Hemorrhagic Septicemia Disease. Genome Announcements 2(4) · July 2014
3. Ahir, V.B., A. Roy, M. K. Jhala, B. B. Bhanderi, R. A. Mathakiya, V. D. Bhatt, K. B. Padiya, S. J. Jakhesara, P. G. Koringa, and C. G. Joshi (2011) Genome Sequence of *Pasteurella multocida* subsp. *gallicida*Anand1_poultry. J. Bacteriol. 193(19) : 5604.
4. Anon. Haemorrhagic septicaemia. In : OIE Manual of Diagnostic Tests and Vaccines for Terrestrial Animals. 2012; Chapter 2.4. 12, pp 1v13.
5. Bain, R,V.S. (1963). Haeamorrhagic septicaemia. FAO Agricultural Studies. Monograph No. 62. Food and Agriculture Organization of the United Nations, Rome, 1963.
6. Boycce, J.D. and Adler, B. (2000) The capsule is a virulence determinant in the pathogenesis of Pasteurella multocida M1404 (B:2). Infect.Immun, 68: 3463-3468].
7. Cao Peili, GuoDongchum, Liu Jiasen, Jiand, Qian, Xu, Zhuofei and Qu, Liandong (2017) Genome-Wide Analyses Reveal Genes Subject to Positive Selection in *Pasteurella multocida.* Front. Microbiol., 30 May 2017 | https://doi.org/10.3389/fmicb.2017.00961.
8. Chhabra Rajesh, R Sharma and N K Kakker (2004). Comparative immunogenecity of Foot and Mouth Disease Virus antigens in.

   FMD-haemorrhagic septicaemia combined vaccine and FMD vaccine alone in buffalo calves. Indian J Exp. Biol. 42: 259-264.
9. Dutta, T.K., Gautam Rajeev, Singh, V.P. and Kumar, A.A. Molecular characterization of India isolates of Psteurella multocida serotype B:2 using REA, RAPD-PCR and ribotyping. Indian J Anim. Sc. 74: 572-576.

10. Kumar, A.A., Shivchandra, S.B., Biswas, A., Singh, V.P., Singh Vijendra P and Srivastava, S.K. (2004) Prevalent Serotypes of *Pasteurella multocida* Isolated from Different Animal and Avian Species in India. Vet. Res. Comm. 2004, 28:657-667.

11. Biswas, A., Shivchandra, S.B., Saxena, M.K., Kumar, A.A., Singh, V.P. and Srivastava, S.K. (2004) Molecular variability among Strains of *Pasteurella multocida* Isolated from an Outbreak of Haemorrha- gicsepticaemia in India. Vet. Res. Comm. 28: 287-298.

12. PallabChaudhuri, V.P.Singh, A Thamizharasan, Jonathan Lalsiamthara (2012) *Pasteurella multocida* P52 aroA mutant conferred protection to rabbits and mice against haemorrhagic septicaemia. DHR Int. J. Biomed Life Sci. 3 (1) : 127-136.

13. Harper, M, Boycee John D and Adler, B. Pasteurella multocida pathogenesis: 125 years after Pasteur. FEMS Microbiol. Lett. 2006, 265-1-10.

14. Horadagoda, N.U., Hodgson, J.C. Moon, G.M., Wijewardana, T.G. and Eckersall, P.D. (2001). Role of endotoxin in the pathogenesis of haemorrhagic septicaemia in the buffalo. Microbial Path. 30:171-178.

15. Khrab S and Charan Shiv, (2013). Mouse model of haemorrha-gicsepticaemia:dissemination and multiplication of Pasteurella multocida B:2 in vital organs after intranasal and subcutaneous challenge in mice. Vet. Res. Commun. 37: 59-63.

16. Kumar, A.A., Shivchandra, S.B., Biswas, A., Singh, V.P., Singh Vijendra P and Srivastava, S.K. (2004) Prevalent serotypes of Pasdteurella multocida Isolated from Different Animal and Avian Species in India. Vet. Res. Commun. 28: 657-667.

17. Liu, Wenjing Liu, Minjun Yang, ZhuofeiXu, HuajunZheng, Wan Liang, Rui Zhou, Bin Wu and Huanchun Chen (2012) Complete Genome Sequence of *Pasteurella multocida* HN06, a Toxigenic Strain of Serogroup D. J. Bact.194, 12: 3292-3293.

18. May, B. J., Zhang, Q., Li, L. L., Paustian, M. L., Whittam, T. S., and Kapur, V. (2001). Complete genomic sequence of *Pasteurella multocida*, Pm70. *Proc. Natl. Acad. Sci. U.S.A.* 98, 3460–3465. doi: 10.1073/pnas.051634598.

19. Moustafa, A. M., Seemann, T., Gladman, S., Adler, B., Harper, M., Boyce, J. D., *et al.* (2015). Comparative genomic analysis of asian Haemorrhagic Septicaemia- associated strains of *Pasteurella multocida* identifies More than 90 Haemorrhagic Septicaemia- Specific Genes. *PLoS ONE* 10:e0130296. doi: 10.1371/journal.pone.0130296.

20. Olson, N.C., Hellyer, P.W. and Dodam, J.R. (1995).Mediators and vascular effects in response to endotoxin. Br. Vet. J. 151:489-522.

21. Othman, Sarah, Parton, R. and Coote John (2012). Interaction between mammalian cells and Pasteurella multocida B:2 Adherence, invasion and intracellular survival. Microbial Path. 52: 353-358.

22. Prasannavadhana , A. , Santosh Kumar, Prasad Thomas, Laxmi Narayan Sarangi, Santosh Kumar Gupta, Adyasha Priyadarshini, Viswas Konasagara Nagaleekar, and Vijendra Pal Singh (2014) Outer Membrane Proteome Analysis of Indian Strain of *Pasteurella multocida* Serotype B:2 by MALDI-TOF/MS Analysis. Scientific World Journal. 2014; 2014: 617034.

23. Priya G. Bhuvana, Viswas Konasagara Nagaleekar, A. Arun Prince Milton, M. Saminathan, Amod Kumar, Amit Ranjan Sahoo, Sajad Ahmad Wani, Amit Kumar, S.K. Gupta, Aditya P. Sahoo, A.K. Tiwari, R.K. Agarwal, Ravi Kumar Gandham (2017). Genome wide host gene expression analysis in mice experimentally infected with Pasteurella multocida. PLoS ONE 12(7): e0179420. https://doi.org/10.1371/journal.pone.0179420.

24. Rimler, R.B. and Rhoades, K.R. (1987) Serogroup F, a new capsule serogroup of *Pasteurella multocida*. J. Clin. MIcrobiol. 25 (4): 615-618.

25. L. N. Sarangi, P. Thomas, S. K. Gupta, S. Kumar, K. N. Viswas, V. P. Singh (2014) Molecular Epidemiology of ***Pasteurella multocida*** Circulating in India by Multilocus Sequence Typing. TransboundaryEmerg Dis. 63(2): 286-292.

26. Saxena, M.K., Singh, V.P., Kumar, A.a., Chaudhari, P., Singh Vijendra Pal, Shivachandra, S.B., Biswas, A. And Sharma, B. (2006) REPO-PCR Analysis of Pasteurella multocidaIsolates from Wild and Domestic Animals in India. Vet. Res. Commun. 30: 851-861.

27. Shivachandra, SathishBhadravati; Kumar, Abhinendra; Yogisharadhya, Revanaiah; Ramakrishnan, M. A.; Viswas, K. N. (2013). Carboxyl terminus heterogeneity of type IV fimbrial subunit protein of Pasteurella multocida isolates. Vet. Res. Commun. 37(4): 269-275.

28. Shivachandra Sathish Bhadravati, Abhinendra Kumar, Nihar Nalini Mohanty, RevanaiahYogisharadhy, NirmalChacko, K.N. Viswas, Muthannan Andavar Ramakrishnan (2014) Homogeneity of VacJ outer membrane lipoproteins among Pasteurella multocida strains and heterogeneity among members of Pasteurel laceae. Res. Vet Sci. 96: 415–421.

29. Singh, Mamta, VermaRishendra, PanditRamaneSangram, TarfainNajeeb UI (2017) Host responses and bacterial colonization following inoculation of ***Pasteurella multocida*** P_{52} strain into unvaccinated and aluminum hydroxide gel hemorrhagic septicemia vaccinated mice. Microbial.Path.

30. Vaid RK, Shanmugasundaram K, Boora A, Bera BC, Shukla BN, Anand T, Singha H, Riyesh T, Virmani N, Barua S, Ahir VB, Koringa PG, Sajnani

MR, Bhat VD, Rana N, Singh KP, Malik P, Singh RK, Joshi CG. 2014. Draft genome sequence of ***Pasteurella multocida*** subsp. ***multocida*** B:2 strain VTCCBAA264 isolated from ***Bubalusbubalis*** in north India. Genome Announc. 2(4):e00755-14. doi:10.1128/genomeA.00755-14.

31. Verma Rishendra and Jaiswal, T.N. (1997) Haemorrhagic septicaemia vaccines. Vaccine 16: 1154-1162.

32. Verma Rishendra (1998) Haemorrhagic septicaemia in buffaloes: Current trends and prophylaxis. Indian J. Anim. Prod. 31: 232-242.

33. VermaHarshit (2013) development and standardization of double emulsified vaccine against swine septic pastuerellosis. Ph.D. Thesis submitted to ICAR-Indian Veterinary Research Institute, Izatnagar-243 122 (Uttar Pradesh), India.

34. Wilson, Brenda A. and Ho, Mengfei (2013) Pasteurella multocida: from Zoonosis to Cellular Microbiology. Clin. Microbiol. Reviews, 26(3): 631-655.

❑❑❑

Chapter 12

Next Generation Sequencing Technology and Its Applications

AMITOZ KOUR[1*], ANIL TAKU[1], S GURDEEP SINGH[2], R.K. SHARMA[3], VIBHA RAJ SHANTI[4], M.A. BHAT[1] AND DIBYENDU CHAKRABORTY[2]

[1] Div. of Veterinary Microbiology, FVSc&AH, SKUAST-J, R.S.Pura, Jammu
[2] Div. AGB, FVSc&AH, SKUAST-J, R.S.Pura, Jammu
[3] Div. ANN, FVSc&AH, SKUAST-J, R.S.Pura, Jammu
[4] School of Biotechnology, SKUAST-J, Chatha *E-mail : amitozkaur78@gmail.com

Introduction

DNA double stranded structure was established by Watson and Crick in the year 1953, but it took more than decades to develop DNA sequencing methods. In 1970, Ray Wu developed the first method to define the DNA sequence using location specific primer extension strategy and therefore, synthetic location - specific primer was used to determine the sequence between the years 1970 and 1973 (Padmanabhan and Wu 1972 ; Wu *et al.*, 1973). Later in 1977 Maxam and Gilbert used Chemical degradation method to sequence DNA. DNA sequencing method with chain-terminating inhibitors was developed by Frederick Sanger, which is now considered as the first generation sequencing method (Sanger *et al.*, 1975) which identifies linear randomly terminated nucleotide sequences, whereas automated Sanger's method uses fluorescent labelled terminators. Out of above all methods, the most accurate, most available and well defined technology is Sanger sequencing method as the throughout of this automated method can read 96 reactions in parallel. Over the past few years, there has been a fundamental shift away from the application of automated Sanger sequencing for genome analysis. Before this, the automated Sanger method had dominated the industry for almost two decades and led to a number of monumental accomplishments, including the completion of the only finished-grade human genome sequence.In spite of many technical improvements during this era, the limitations of automated Sanger sequencing showed a need for new and improved technologies for sequencing large numbers of human genomes. Using this method, complete human genome would take around 60 years to synthesize and costing approximately $5 to 30 million USD. Recent efforts have been directed towards the development of new methods, leaving Sanger sequencing with fewer reported advances. The automated Sanger method is considered as a 'first-generation' technology and recent newer methods are referred to as next-generation sequencing (NGS). Next generation high throughput sequencing technologies are capable of sequencing large number DNA sequences in a single reaction, by using combination of template preparation, sequencing and imaging, along with genome alignment and assembly methods.

The need and demand for low cost sequencing lead to the development of next generation sequencing (high-throughout sequencing) technologies in which these are able to produce an enormous volume of data cheaply and in some cases, in excess of one billion short reads per instrument run. This ability expands the realm of experimentation beyond just determining the order of bases as ingene-expression studies microarrays are now being replaced by sequence-based methods, which can identify and quantify rare transcripts without having prior knowledge of a particular gene and also provide information regarding alternative splicing and sequence variation in identified genes. This capabilityto sequence the whole genome of many related organisms has allowed large-scale comparative and evolutionary studies to be performed that were unimaginable few years ago. The most advantageous application of NGS will be the re-sequencing of human genomes in-order to increase our understanding of how genetic differences can affect health and disease conditions.

Next-Generation Sequencing Technologies

Next generation sequencing technology includes a number of methods that constitutes template preparation, sequencing, imaging and data analysis. One technology differs from other on the basis of combination of specific protocols, which determines the type of data produced from each platform.

For NGS reactions, there are two methods which are used in preparing templates : Clonally amplified templates originating from single DNA molecules and single DNA molecule templates. Other method is sequencing by synthesis (DNA polymerase-dependent methods), which are classified as cyclic reversible termination (CRT), single-nucleotide addition (SNA) and real-time sequencing. The voluminous data produced by these NGS platforms place substantial demands on information technology in terms of data storage, tracking and quality control.

In the template preparation genomic DNA is broken into smaller sizes from which either fragment templates or mate-pair templates are created. A common step among NGS technologies is that the template is attached or immobilized to a solid surface or support and the immobilization of spatially separated template sites allows thousands to billions of sequencing reactions to be performed simultaneously.

Clonally amplified templates are prepared by two most common methods, which include emulsion PCR (emPCR) and solid-phase amplification. EmPCR is used to prepare sequencing templates in a cell-free system,which prevent the arbitrary loss of genomic sequences, that is a major problem in bacterial cloning methods. A library of fragment or mate-pair targets is created, and adaptors containing universal priming sites are ligated to the target ends, allowing complex genomes to be amplified with common PCR primers. After ligation, the DNA is separated into single strands and captured onto beads so that one DNA molecule is attached to each bead. After amplification and enrichment of emPCR beads, millions can be immobilized in a polyacrylamide gel on a standard microscope slide (Polonator)11, chemically crosslinked to an aminocoated glass surface (Life/APG; Polonator)12 or deposited into individual PicoTiterPlate (PTP) wells (Roche/454)13, in which the NGS can be performed.

Solid-phase amplification can also be used to produce clonally amplified clusters from fragment or mate-pair templates on a glass slide. In this type of amplification high-density forward and reverse primers are covalently attached to the slide, and the ratio of the primers to the template on the support defines the surface density of the amplified clusters. Solid-phase amplification produces 100–200 million spatially separated template clusters (Illumina/Solexa), providing free ends to whicha universal sequencing primer can be hybridized to initiate the NGS reaction.

Now-a-days, different NGS Technologies includes 454 pyrosequencing, llumina (Solexa) sequencing, SOLiD Sequencing, Massively parallel signature sequencing (MPSS), Polony sequencing, Ion Torrent semi-conductor sequencing, DNA nanoball sequencing, Heliscope single molecule sequencing and Single molecule real time (SMRT) sequencing which are explained in details below.

1. 454 Pyrosequencing

454 pyrosequencing was first reported in 1988 using the principle of pyrophosphate detection and the technique was further developed (Ronaghi *et al.*, 1996) in Stockholm to analyze 96 samples in parallel in a microtiter plate. In this 454 Genome Sequencer FLX instrument was introduced in 2005 by 454 Life Sciences, which is based on principle of sequencing by synthesis. In this method, the template DNA is ligated with specific adapter to attach one fragment of DNA to a single primer coated on streptavidin bead to form a clonal colony and then Emulsion PCR is carried out with water droplets in an oil solution. The droplets act as individual amplification reactors producing approximately 10^7 clonal copies per bead (Margulies *et al.*, 2005). ATP sulfurylase and luciferase enzymes generate visible light upon incorporation of the complementary nucleotide thus acting as sensors. The amplified DNA is transferred into a picotiter plate which allows hundreds and thousands of parallel pyrosequencing reactions to be carried out increasing the sequencing throughput. This technology measures the release of inorganic pyrophosphate detected by light enzyme luciferase (Tawfik and Griffiths 1998; Nyren *et al.*, 1993) and the light intensity is proportional to the pyro-phosphate released.

2. Illumina (Solexa) Sequencing

This NGS technology was invented by Balasubramanian and Klennerman from Cambridge University's chemistry department. Illumina (Solexa) sequencing is based on reversible dye-terminators technology along with engineered polymerases (Bentley *et al.*, 2008). This method is similar to Sanger sequencing, but uses modified dNTP's con-taining a terminator, which blocks further polymerization. In this Technique DNA molecules (single stranded) are attached to an immobilized surface by an adapter and hybridized to complementary adapters for synthesis of their complementary strands and after the amplification, the templates are sequenced in a massive parallel form using sequencing-by-synthesis approach. To determine the sequence, four types of reversible terminator bases (RT-bases) are added in presence of special DNA poly-merases and then, camera takes images of the fluorescently labelled terminator nucleotides along with its position. Later, the dye along with the terminal 3′ blocker, are chemically removed from the DNA, allowing for the next cycle to begin. The method is highly accurate base by base sequencing by eliminating errors.

3. SOLiD sequencing

In SOLiD sequencing a library of DNA fragments are first ligated to magnetic bead with universal P1 adapter and after that Emulsion PCR takes place in micro-reactors with all reagents of PCR. The resulting beads, each containing single copies of the same DNA molecule, are deposited on a glass slide (Valouev *et al.*, 2008). Now, One DNA fragment per bead bound to an adapter is hybridized with a primer and then, these templates are characterized by fluorescent labels for detection by fluorescence. The sequencing process is again continued in the same way with another primer. Sequences are determined in parallel for more than 50 million bead clusters, resulting in a very high throughput of the order of Giga-bases per run. The new SOLiD instrument is capable of producing 1-3GB of sequence in 8-day run and offers 99.94% accuracy.

4. Ion Torrent Sequencing

Technology is based on semiconductor based detection system. This method of sequencing detects the hydrogen ions that are released during the polymerisation of DNA, as opposite to the optical methods used in other sequencing systems. A microwell containing a template DNA strand to be sequenced is flooded with a single type of nucleotide and If the introduced nucleotide is complementary to the leading template nucleotide, it is incorporated into the growing complementary strand. This causes the release of a hydrogen ion that triggers a hypersensitive ion sensor, which indicates that a reaction has occurred. If homopolymer repeats are present in the template sequence, multiple nucleotides will be incorporated in a single cycle leading to a corresponding number of released hydrogens and a proportionally higher electronic signal (Rusk 2011).

5. Massively Parallel Signature Sequencing (MPSS)

The MPSS was developed in the 1990s at Lynx Therapeutics by Sydney Brenner and Sam Eletr. MPSS is a procedure used for identifying and quantifying mRNA transcripts, which was a bead-based method that used a complex approach of adapter ligation followed by adapter decoding, reading the sequence in increments of four nucleotides. In this mRNA is reverse transcribed into cDNA, cDNA is amplified in microreactors as emulsion PCR. A sequence signature of ~16-20bp is determined from all the beads in parallel. Each signature sequence is cloned onto microbeads and then arrayed in a flow cell for sequencing and quantification. This method made it susceptible to sequence-specific bias or loss of specific sequences.

6. Polony Sequencing

Polony sequencing was developed in the laboratory of George M Church at Harvard and this technique was among the first next-generation sequencing systems, which was used to sequence a full genome in 2005. It combined an *in vitro* paired-tag library with emulsion PCR, an automated microscope, and ligation-based sequencing. The chemistry to sequence an *E. coli* genome at an accuracy of >99.9999% costed approximately 1/9 that of Sanger sequencing (Shendure *et al.*, 2005). Emulsion PCR isolates individual DNA molecules along with primer-coated beads in aqueous droplets within an oil phase. PCR then coats each bead with clonal copies of the DNA molecule followed by immobilization for later sequencing.

7. Heliscope Single Molecule Sequencing

Heliscope sequencing is a method of single-molecule sequencing developed by Helicos Biosciences. This method helps in direct sequencing of cellular and extra-cellular nucleic acids in an unbiased manner. It uses DNA fragments with added poly-A tail adapters, which are attached to the flow cell surface. The next steps involve extension-based sequencing with cyclic washes of the flow cell with fluorescently labeled nucleotides (one nucleotide type at a time, as with the Sanger method). The reads are short, up to 55 bases per run but recent improvements allow for more accurate reads of stretches of one type of nucleotides (Thompson and Steinmann 2010). This sequencing method and equipment were used to sequence the genome of the M13 bacteriophage (Harris *et al.*, 2008).

8. Single Molecule Real Time (SMRT) Sequencing

SMRT sequencing is based on sequencing by synthesis approach. The DNA is synthesized in zero-mode wave-guides (ZMWs) - small well-like containers with the capturing tools located at the bottom of the well. The sequencing is performed with use of unmodified polymerase (attached to the ZMW bottom) and fluorescently labelled nucleotides flowing freely in the solution. The wells are constructed in a way that only the fluorescence occurring by the bottom of the well is detected. The fluorescent label is detached from the nucleotide at its incorporation into the DNA strand, leaving an unmodified DNA strand. According to Pacific Biosciences, the SMRT technology developer, this methodology allows detection of nucleotide modifications (such as cytosine methylation). This happens through the observation of polymerase kinetics. This approach allows reads of 20,000 nucleotides or more, with average read lengths of 5 kilobases. The comparison of major NGS technologies is shown in Table 1.

Table 1. Comparison of Sequencing Technologies Platforms:

NGS Technology	Approach	Read length	Reads per run	Time per run	Cost per 1 million bases
SMRT(Single molecule real time seque-ncing)	sequencing by synthesis (polymerase kinetics)	≥ 40,000 bases	500-1000 Mega bases	30 m to 4h	$ 0.13 t0.60
Ion Semi-conductor (Ion Torrent sequencing	Based on semi-conductor system (hydrogen ion detection)	Upto 400 bp	80 million	2 hours	$1
454/Roche FLX system	Pyrosequen-cing on Solid Support	750 bp	1 million	24 hours	$10
llumina/ solexa	Sequencing by synthesis reversible with Terminators	300- 500 bp	3 million	1-10 days (depending on sequence and specific read length)	$0.05 to 0.12
ABI/ Solid	Massively Parallel seque -ncing by ligation	32 to 50 bp	1.2 to1.4 billions	1 to 2 weeks	$0.13

Applications of Next Generation Sequencing

The production of large numbers of low-cost reads makes the NGS platforms useful for many applications. These include variant discovery by re-sequencing targeted regions of interest or wholegenomes, *de novo* assemblies of bacterial and lower eukaryotic genomes, cataloguing the transcriptomes of cells, tissues and organisms (RNA–seq), genome-wide profiling of epigenetic marks and chromatin structure using other seq-based methods (ChIP–seq, methyl–seq and DNase–seq), and gene discovery by metagenomics studies.

Transcriptome Sequencing

Genome survey of gene expression levels were studied using qPCR, SAGE and microarray with a lot of limitations. Next generation sequencing techniques were implemented along with SAGE tags to sequence the RNA populations from the cells expressed. Noncoding RNA (ncRNA) are any RNA's that are transcribed and not translated to a protein, and these havean important role in regulation of gene expression in plants and animals. These ncRNA are unique, diverse and regulate genes by a variety of mechanisms. Next-generation sequencing technology has discovered many novel ncRNAs (Sanger and Coulson 1975; Gowda*et al.,* 2006; Mardis, 2006). The readouts from next generation technologies are quantitative, allowing to detect changes in expression levels due to changes in environment and onset of disease.Remarkable progress has been made in characterizing and understanding these molecules using next generation technologies, which may help in uncover certain aspects of disease or cancer. Discovering ncRNAs and sequencing of transcriptome would provide us new insights on the genome wide expression patterns of an organism.

Resurrection ofAncient Genomes

With the advent of molecular techniques, such as PCR and DNA sequencing, deciphering of mitochondrial genomes from fossils and ancient remnants was possible. These samples are easily degraded as well as several complications arose from these cases, mainly DNA contamination. Next generation sequencing can be implemented to obtain sequence information from the degraded nature of the ancient genome. Sequence information from single fossil bone of Neanderthal genome was obtained using next generation sequencing technologies

(Carrilho 2000). In addition to Neanderthal sequence, information was also obtained directly from the nuclear genomes of ancient remains of the cave bear (Robertson *et al.*, 2007) and mammoth (Barski *et al.*, 2007). In this way next - generation sequencing technology can be used in resurrecting ancient genomes.

Analysis of Epigenetic Modifications of Histones and DNA

Next -generation sequencing technologies made it possible to study DNA methylation profile by bisulphite DNA sequencing, mapping histone modifications, mapping the locations of DNA-binding proteins, DNA accessibility and chromatin structure. The association between DNA and proteins is an interaction regulating gene expression and controlling the availability of DNA for transcription, replication, and other processes. Genome-wide chromatin immunoprecipitation (ChIP)-based studies for DNA-protein interactions became possible in sequenced genomes (Korbel *et al.*, 2007). ChIP-based approach and the Illumina platform provided insights into transcription factor binding sites in the human genome, such as neuron-restrictive silencer factor (NRSF) (Tawfik and Griffiths 1998) and signal transducer and activator of transcription 1 (STAT1) (Bhinge *et al.*, 2007). So, next generation sequencing technologies can be used for understanding of gene expression–based cellular responses due to DNA-protein interactions.

Sequence Census Applications

The large numbers of short reads produced by next-generation sequencers provide opportunities for the development of new applications that benefit from the particular data format. For instance, next-generation technologies have been widely applied in contexts, whereby sequencing of only a portion of the molecule is sufficient (referred to assequence census applications). The sequence census approach uses short reads (or "tags") to assign the site of origin of the read instead of determining the entire sequence of the original DNA molecule. By mapping the sequence read to its molecule of origin, the presence of the molecule is established. Significantly, the number of reads that map to a particular nucleic acid species correlates with the abundance of the species in the cell.

Human Genome Studies

In October 2007, venter and colleagues described the genome sequence of J. Craigventer using a whole-genome shotgun (venter *et al.,* 2007) approach coupled with automated Sanger sequencing. Human genome studies aim to catalogue SNVs and SVs and their association to phenotypic differences, with the eventual goal of personalized genomics for medical purposes. The first group to apply NGS to whole human genomes was Roche/454 in collaboration with Gibbs and colleagues at the BCM-HGSC, who reported the diploid genome of James D. watson. After compairing the watson genome with the reference genome (Publised on NCBI), roughly 3.3 million SNVs were identified, but far fewer SVs were found than in the study by venterand colleagues. This is important because undiscovered SVs could account for a substantial fraction ofthe total number of sequence variants, many of which could be potentially causative in disease.

Conclusion

Next-generation sequencing approaches are poised to emerge as the dominant genomics technology due to their much improved cost effectiveness, compared to Sanger sequencing. In addition to the applications described above, NGS technologies are being used to characterize the evolutionary relationships of ancient genomes and to elucidate the role of non-coding RNAs in health and disease. In future, it is foreseeable that NGS technologies could be used to obtain high-quality sequence data froma genome isolated from a single cell, which would be a substantial breakthrough, particularly for cancer genomics. The field of NGS technology is a fast-moving area of research,which makes this an exciting time for genomic studies.

References

Barski A, S Cuddapah, K Cui, T Y Roh, D E Schones, Z Wang, G Wei, I Chepelev and K. Zhao. 2007. High-resolution profiling of histone methylations in the human genome. *Cell.*129: 823–37.

Bentley D R, S Balasubramanian, H P Swerdlow, G P Smith and J Milton. 2008. Accurate whole human genome sequencing using reversible terminator chemistry. *Nature* : 456 (7218) : 53-59.

Bhinge A A, J Ki, G M Euskirche, M Snyder and V RIyer. 2007. Mapping the chromo-somal targets of STAT1 by sequence tag analysis of genomic enrichment (STAGE). *Genome Research.* 17 : 910–916.

Carrilho E. 2000. DNA sequencing by capillary array electrophoresis and microfabricated array systems. *Electrophoresis*.21 : 55–65.

Gowda M, H Li, J Alessi, F Chen, R Pratt and G L Wang. 2006. Robust analysis of 5¢-transcript ends (5¢-RATE) : a novel technique for transcriptome analysis and genome annotation. *Nucleic Acids Research*. 34 : e126.

Harris T D, P R Buzby, H Babcock, E Beer, J Bowers and I Braslavsky. 2008. Single-molecule DNA sequencing of a viral genome. *Science* 320 (5872) : 106–109.

Korbel J O, A E Urban, J P Affourtit, B Godwin, F Grubert, J F Simons, P M Kim, D Palejev, N J Carriero, L Du, B E Taillon, Z Chen, A Tanzer, A C Saunders, J Chi, F Yang, N P Carter, M E Hurles, S M Weissman, T T Harkins, M B Gerstein, M Egholm and M Snyder. 2007. Paired-end mapping reveals extensive structural variation in the human genome. *Science*. 318 : 420–26.

Mardis E R. 2006. Anticipating the 1,000 dollar genome. *Genome Biology*. 7 : 112.

Margulies M , M Egholm, W E Altman, S Attiya and J S Bader. 2005. Genome sequencing in microfabricated high-density picolitre reactors. *Nature*. 437 : 376–80.

Nyren P, B Pettersson and MUhlen. 1993. Solid phase DNA minisequencing by an enzymatic luminometric inorganic pyrophosphate detection assay. *Analytical Biochemistry*. 208. 171–75.

Padmanabhan R, R Wu and E Jay. 1972. Chemical synthesis of a primer and its use in the sequence analysis of the lysozyme gene of bacteriophage T4. *Proceedings of National Academy of Science*. 71 (6) : 2510–14.

Robertson G, M Hirst, M Bainbridge, M Bilenky, Y Zhao, T Zeng, G Euskirchen, B Bernier, R Varhol, A Delaney, N Thiessen, O L Griffith, A H M. Marra, M Snyder and S Jones. 2007. Genome-wide profiles of STAT1 DNA association using chromatin immunoprecipitation and massively parallel sequencing. *Nature Methods*. 4 : 651–657

Ronaghi M, SKaramohamed, B Pettersson, MUhlen, and P. Nyren. 1996. Real-time DNA sequencing using detection of pyrophosphate release. *Analytical Biochemistry*. 242 : 84–89.

Rusk N. 2011. Torrents of sequence. *Nature Methods*. 8 (1) : 44–44.

Sanger F, and A R Coulson. 1975. A rapid method for determining sequences in DNA by primed synthesis with DNA polymerase. *Journal of Molecular Biology*. 94 : 441–448.

Shendure J, G J Porreca, N B Reppas, X Lin, J P McCutcheon, A M Rosenbaum, M D Wang, K Zhang, R D Mitra and G M. Church. 2005. Accurate multiplex polony sequencing of an evolved bacterial genome. *Science*. 309 (5741) : 1728–1732.

Tawfik D S and A D Griffiths. 1998. Man-made cell-like compartments for molecular evolution. *Natural Biotechnology*. 16 : 652–656.

Thompson J F and K E Steinmann. 2010. Single molecule sequencing with a HeliScope genetic analysis system. *Current Protocols in Molecular Biology*. Chapter 7 : Unit7.10.

Venter J C, K Remington, J F Heidelberg, A L Halpern, D Rusch, and J A Eisen. 2007. Environmental genome shotgun sequencing of the Sargasso Sea. *Science*. 304 (5667) : 66-74.

Valouev A, J Ichikawa, T Tonthat, J Stuart, S Ranade, and H Peckham. 2008. A high-resolution, nucleosome position map of *C. elegans*reveals a lack of universal sequence-dictated positioning. *Genome Research*. 18 (7) : 1051–1063.

Wu R, C D Tu and R Padmanabhan. 1973. Nucleotide sequence analysis of DNA. XII. The chemical synthesis and sequence analysis of a dodecadeoxynucleotide, which binds to the endolysin gene of bacteriophage lambda. *Biophysics Research Communication*. 55(**4**) : 1092–99.

□□□

Chapter 13

Designer Milk for Human Health : A Future Need

ARVIND KUMAR* SAKSHI SHARMA* AND DHIRENDER KUMAR**

* Division of Livestock Products Technology, F.V.Sc. &A.H., R.S. Pura, SKUAST-Jammu

** Division of Animal Genetics and Breeding, F.V.Sc. &A.H., R.S. Pura, SKUAST-Jammu

Introduction

Recent evidences of epidemiological linkages between diet and chronic diseases have prompted the search for new clinical insights into the relationship between food and the onset (or prevention) of disease. In this context, the extra-nutritional therapeutic attributes of milk and milk products are no longer debated. Advances in biotechnology and genetic engineering have hinted at possibilities that were hitherto not fathomed in the field of dairying. It is now firmly established that a new generation of value-added products can be harvested from milk and milk products. While until recently, emphasis has been on breeding large animals to produce more milk, the attention is now tuned to adding more value to milk and studying its health implications. Milk composition can be altered by nutritional management or through the exploitation of naturally occurring genetic variation among cattle. By a thorough understanding of the biochemistry, genetic traits and changes in the cow's diet that affect milk synthesis and composition, ways and means to manipulate milk composition to suit specific needs can be found. By combining the two approaches of nutritional and genetic interventions, researchers are now hoping to develop 'designer milk' tailored to consumer preferences or rich in specific milk components that have implications in health as well as processing. This article exposes the readers to the potential that exists in altering the milk composition or 'designing' milk by nutritional and genetic approaches so as to achieve specific health and/or processing opportunities.

Opportunities of 'Designing' Milk

Milk is an ingredient that is consumed globally. The current interests, processing and research-wise are the healthful and therapeutic aspects of milk and milk products. To realize the full potential of these advantages, it would be desirable to have the opportunity to alter milk composition in several ways. For diet and human health measures, the actions that would be beneficial are:

a) Generate a greater proportion of unsaturated fatty acids (USFA) in milk fat.

b) Reduce lactose content in milk in order to cater to persons suffering from lactose intolerance.

c) Remove b-lactoglobulin (b-lg) from milk.

From a technological point of view, there exist vast opportunities in:

a) Alteration of primary structure of casein to improve technological properties of milk.

b) Production of high-protein milk.

c) Engineering milk meant for cheese manufacturing that leads to accelerated curd clotting time.

d) Increased yield and/or more protein recovery.

e) Milk containing nutraceuticals.

f) Replacement for infant formula.

Modifications in Protein

One of the major products of the mammary glands being protein, exciting research and technology opportunities extend the frontiers for better protein supplementation. Improved amino acid profile by the addition of L-taurine, L-leucine and L-phenylalanine offers additional nutritional benefits.

Transgenic cows secreting elevated levels of b-(8–20%) and k-caseins (twofold) have been produced by genetic engineering(1). b-casein, which is the most abundant milk protein, is involved in binding calcium phosphate and thus, controlling milk calcium levels.

Higher k-casein content in milk is linked to smaller micelles, better heat stability, and improved cheese-making properties. In the transgenic animals engineered by Brophy's group, the total milk protein increased by 13–20% and total milk casein by 17-35% compared to non-transgenic control cows. This has obviously, a positive influence on the cheese yield and also on the casein and milk protein concentrate industry.

Edible casein is used in vitamin tablets, instant drinks and infant formulas, whereas acid casein is used for paper coatings, cosmetics, button making, paints and textile fabrics (2). Caseins, particularly the b-, as1- and as2-caseins, being easily digestible are quite sensitive to plasmin, a serine protease occurring naturally in milk along with plasminogen. Plasmin activity leads to limited proteolysis in milk. This offers a dual disadvantage of decreasing the curd yield in cheese and inducing organoleptic defects and gelation of ultra high temperature-treated milk. Milk augmented with specific inhibitors of either plasmin or plaminogen activator would, therefore, be a boon to the process industry (3).

A2 Milk TM from commercial dairy herds is being marketed in New Zealand and Australia at a small premium over regular or A1 milk. A2 Corporation scientists claim that as A2 Milk TM has only negligible amounts of the A1 b casein in it, the perceived risks associated with the consumption of this type of casein (such as autism or Asperger's syndrome, child diabetes, schizophrenia and coronary heart disease) are effectively removed (4).

They further maintain that A2 b-casein was the original b-casein gene, whereas subsequent genetic mutation generated A1 b-casein. Hence, all milk produced by cattle thousands of years ago, before the large-scale domestication of cows, was A2 Milk TM. The animals producing A2 Milk TM are not genetically modified. It is achieved by selectively milking only those cows that naturally produce milk without AI.

Modifications in Fat

The 'ideal' milk fat for human health would contain < 10% poly unsaturated fatty acids (PUFA), < 8% saturated fatty acids (SFA), and > 82% monosaturated fatty acids(5). Although it may not be possible to achieve this 'ideal' milk fat composition, manipulation of composition of milk fat is possible through altering the feeding practices for dairy cows and also through genetic interventions. Decreasing the level of saturation in milk fat feeding of unsaturated fats in an encapsulated or protected form results in a prompt rise in the degree of unsaturation of the serum lipids, tissue fat and milk fat6.

Feeding highly unsaturated oils (e.g. soybean oil) caused depression in milk fat, but increased the proportion of USFA to SFA in milk . A study at the University of Alberta (7) revealed that feeding canola oil in the encapsulated form (to protect it from biohydrogenation by the rumen micro-organisms) led to higher increases in linoleic (18 : 2) and linolenic (18 : 3) acids than while feeding unprotected oil seeds. As the melting point of milk fat containing USFA is more, the spreadability of butter made from this milk improved tremendously.

An Australian study involving the feeding of a special blend of canola and soybean meal in the protected form resulted in doubling in the spreadability of butter(8) . When taken out of a fridge at 5°C, the butter was nearly as spreadable as margarine, without losing its special eating qualities. Clinical trials revealed that consumption of dairy products made from this milk led to decrease in LDL levels in the blood of the consumers.

Studies at the University of California (Davis) are focused on the desaturase gene to produce milk with decreased levels of SFA (9). Efforts are underway to determine, if genetic differences among breeds and individual animals are translated into ratios of SFA and USFA. Increasing conjugated linoleic acid levels in milk fat Dairy products are rich in conjugated linoleic acid (CLA), a product synthesized in the rumen during the biohydrogenation of linoleic acid.

A diet rich in linoleic acid led to increasing the CLA levels in milk fat twofold (10). Incorporating CLA along with soy oil in the diet of cows increased the CLA levels, simultaneously decreasing the SFA in milk fat (11). Furthermore, milk from a grass-fed cow can have five times as much CLA as milk from a grain-fed animal.

CLAs reportedly suppress carcinogens, inhibiting proliferation of leukaemia and cancers of the colon, prostate, ovary and breast. They are the only natural fatty acids accepted by the National Academy of Sciences, USA as exhibiting consistent antitumour properties at levels as low as 0.25–1.0% of total fats (12). The other reported beneficial health effects of CLA, as supported by biomedical studies with animal models are anti-atherogenic effect, altered nutrient partitioning and lipid metabolism, antidiabetic action (type II diabetes), immunity enhancement and improved bone mineralization (13).

The 9,11 isomer of CLA in milk fat is synthesized by the cow and not rumen bacteria. Synthesis involves a mammary enzyme, delta-9 desaturase, which acts on a trans-fatty (vaccenic) acid produced by rumen bacteria. Several genetic factors that regulate the expression of the delta-9 desaturase gene have been identified.

Reducing Fat Content in Milk

As a variation to altering the fat composition, the modification in cow's genetic makeup to enable it to produce milk with 2% fat would reduce the cost of feed per kg milk by 22% (15). In changing the fat composition, targeting enzymes that influence the synthesis of fat is important. As an example, reduction of acetyl CoA carboxylase that regulates the rate of fat synthesis within the mammary gland would translate to a drastic reduction in the fat content of milk and reduce the energy required by the animal to produce milk (16).

Type of fatty acids vs product quality

The type of fatty acids present in milk fat can influence the flavour and physical properties of dairy products. There are reports that butter produced from cows fed with high oleic sunflower seeds and regular sunflower seeds were equal or superior in flavour to the control butter (17).

The experimental butter was softer, more unsaturated and exhibited acceptable flavour, manufacturing, and storage characteristics. Extruded soyabean and sunflower diets yielded Cheddar cheese that had higher concentration of USFA while maintaining flavour, manufacturing and storage characteristics similar to that of control cheese (18). It is also beneficial from a safety point of view, as the accumulation of fatty acids, namely C12, C14, C18: 1 and C18: 2 enhanced the safety of cheese against *Listeria monocytogenes* and *Salmonella typhimurium* (19).

Humanization of Bovine Milk

It is said that mother's breast milk is the ultimate designer food for babies. However, due to varying reasons, a number of infants are fed formulas based on bovine milk. The composition of these formulas could be greatly improved to suit the needs of the infant by incorporation of ingredients that resemble those of human milk, thereby 'humanizing' the bovine milk.

Lactoferrin (LF), the iron-binding protein has antimicrobial properties and may also mediate some effects of inflammation and have a role in regulating various components of the immune system. Its level in human milk is about 1 g/l (in human colostrum about 7 g/l). As the levels of LF in cow's milk is only about one-tenth that in human milk, this has caught the attention of those involved in designing human milk replacement formulas. Pharming, NV (Leiden, The Netherlands) developed the first transgenic bull in the late 1980s and a line of transgenic cows to produce several proteins, including human LF (hLF) (20).

Human milk contains 0.4 g/l of lysozyme (LZ), an enzyme that provides it with antibacterial activity. Active human lysozyme (hLZ) has been produced in the milk of transgenic mice at concentrations of 0.78 g/l (21). On the processing front, the expression of LZ in milk results in the reduction of rennet clotting time and greater gel strength in the clot. A double transgenic cow that co-expresses both, hLF and hLZ in milk may also reduce the incidence of intra-mammary infection or mastitis.

Yet another application of transgenic technology could be to produce the human lipase, which is stimulated by bile salt in the milk of bovines. The lipase thus produced could be used as a constituent of formulas to increase the digestibility of lipids, especially in premature infants who have low b-gal activity (22). From a study involving African-Americans between the ages 12 and 40 years, Johnson et al.(23) concluded that the cause of milk intolerance in as many as one-third of the subjects claiming symptoms after ingestion of a moderate amounts of milk was not its lactose content.

Cow milk allergenicity in children is often caused by the presence of b-lg, which is absent in human milk. Elimination of this protein by knocking out b-lg gene from cow's milk is unlikely to have any detrimental effects on either cow or human formula and might actually overcome many of the major allergy problems associated with cow's milk. Further, as milk protein allergenicity studies demonstrate that all food proteins are potential allergens and that allergenic structures are widely spread throughout the protein molecule, milk is a good model in the search for means of characterizing allergenic structures in food (24). Therefore, while developing strategies for the identification and evaluation of potential allergenicity in novel foods, many of the technological practices used in the assessment of milk protein allergenicity can be adapted.

Milk with Human Therapeutic Proteins

Industrial interest has focused on the production of high value, low volume therapeutic proteins in the milk of domestic animals. In this context, several human proteins have already been expressed with success. GTC Biotherapeutics (Framingham, MA) uses both, goats and cows to produce more than 60 therapeutic proteins, including plasma proteins, monoclonal antibodies and vaccines.

One product that is in late stages of testing is recombinant human antithrombin III (produced in goat milk), an anti-coagulant protein found in blood. GTC is also working on a project to develop a malaria vaccine from goat milk. It is understood that a litre of goat milk can contain up to 9 g of the transgenic protein and that eight goats can produce enough vaccine to inoculate 20 million people.

The cost to produce a transgenic protein in goat milk can thus be 3 to 30 times cheaper than the current method using mammalian cell culture. PPL Therapeutics (Edinburgh, UK and Blacksburg, VA) is working with rabbits and sheep to produce a-1-antitrypsin, fibrinogen, and a lipase to treat pancreatic insufficiency in digesting dietary lipids. Products, such as insulin and growth hormone have also been obtained from the milk of transgenic cows, sheep or goats.

The Future

Mice that produce milk with 33% more total solids (40– 50% TS) and 17% less lactose than normal control mice have been generated by transgene. As the increase in the TS is associated with a decrease in total milk volume, the same amount of total milk fat and protein is being produced in a lesser total milk volume. If this technology could be propagated in dairy animals, milk that contains 6.5% protein, 7% fat, 2.5% lactose and 50% less water is not an improbable accomplishment. The advantages would be (a) direct economic benefit in terms of 50% reduction in the cost of shipping milk, (b) less stress on the cow and on her udder, since the cow would be producing one-half her normal volume of milk, (c) skim milk with twice protein content and half the lactose content of normal milk, (d) easier to produce low lactose or lactose-free dairy products, (e) better product yields due to concentration, (f) reduction in total whey output because of low milk volume and lactose content and (g) decrease in mastitis as less lactose available for organisms.

Despite all these promising prospects, there is a tendency among human beings to resist change, especially those that trouble their feeling and instincts. As all changes that arise as a consequence of biological research would fall into these categories, there is bound to be tremendous resistance to topics, such as transgenics. The future of biotechnologically derived foods is, therefore, at crossroads even after two decades of positive results. Hi-tech milk processing may be more acceptable to consumers than transgenesis for altering milk composition. Controversy will inevitably tint all biotechnological manipulations aimed at increasing milk production or altering milk composition. Ultimate acceptability will depend on the four key factors of animal welfare, demonstrable safety of the product, enhanced health properties of the product and increased profitability compared with conventional practices. Various ethical, legal and social aspects of biotechnological research need to be addressed before we would see designer transgenic herds similar to the organic herds that thrive in the current economic and social climate.

References

1. Brophy, B., Smolenski, G., Wheeler, T., Wells, D., L'Huillier, P. and Laible, G., Cloned transgenic cattle produce milk with higher levels of beta-casein and kappa-casein. *Nature Biotechnol.*, 2003, 21, 157–162.
2. Karatzas, C. N., Designer milk from transgenic clones. *Nature Biotechnol.*, 2003, 21, 138–139.
3. Murthy, G. L. N. and Kanawjia, S. K., Designer milk: Nutritional and technological significance. *Indian Dairyman*, 2002, 54, 49–58
4. Lacefield, G. D., Designer milk. Forage News, 2003; www.uky.edu
5. O'Donnel, J. A., Milk fat technologies and markets: A summary of the Wisconsin Milk Marketing Board 1988 Milk Fat Roundtable. *J. Dairy Sci.*, 1989, 72, 3109–3115.
6. Ashes, J. R., Gulati, S. K. and Scott, T. W., Potential to alter content and composition of milk fat through nutrition. *J. Dairy Sci.*, 1997, 80, 2204–2212.
7. Mason, S., Manipulating milk composition. ProLivestock, 2001, www.afns.ualberta.ca

8. CSIRO Media Release, Healthy butter spreads better. 1999; www.csiro.au

9. California Dairy Research Foundation, Investigators aim to improve milk composition for increased utilization. *Pre-harvest Research*, 2004; www.cdrf.org/newsletter

10. Beaulieu, A. D. and Drackley, J. K., Can milk fat be beneficial to your health? Illini DairyNet. The Online Resource for the Dairy Industry, 2004; www.traill.uiuc.edu

11. Pszczola, D. E., Katz, F. and Giese, J., Research trends in healthful foods. *Food Technol.*, 2000, 54, 45–52.

12. Eynard, A. R. and Lopez, C. B., Conjugated linoleic acid (CLA) versus saturated fats/cholesterol: their proportion in fatty and lean meats may affect the risk of developing colon cancer. *Lipids Health Dis.*, 2003, 2, 6, www.pubmedcentral.nih.gov.htm

13. Bauman, D. E., Corl, B. A., Baumgard, L. H. and Griinari, J. M., Conjugated linoleic acid (CLA) and the dairy cow. In Recent Advances in Animal Nutrition-2001 (eds Garnsworthy, P. C. and Wiseman, J.), Nottingham University Press, Nottingham, UK, 2001, pp. 221–250.

14. Bauman, D. E. and Perfield, J. W. II, CLA – the milk fat wonder. Pro-dairy. *North East Dairy Business*, 2002, 6, 21, (www.dairybusiness.com)

15. Wall, R. J., Keer, D. E. and Bondioli, K. R., Transgenic dairy cattle: Genetic engineering on a large scale. *J. Dairy Sci.*, 1997, 80, 2213–2224.

16. Ntambi, J. M., Choi, Y. and Kim, Y. C., Regulation of stearoylCoA desaturase by conjugated linoleic acid. In Advances in Conjugated Linoleic Acid Research (eds Yurawecz, M. P. et al.), AOCS Press, Champaign, USA, 1999, vol. 1, pp. 340–347.

17. Middaugh, R. P., Bear, R. J., Casper, D. P., Schingoethe, D. J. and Seas, S. W., Characteristics of milk and butter from cows fed sunflower seeds. *J. Dairy Sci.*, 1988, 71, 3179–3187.

18. Lightfield, K. K., Bear, R. J. and Schingoethe, D. J., Characteristics of milk and Cheddar cheese from cows fed unsaturated dietary fat. *J. Dairy Sci.*, 1993, 76, 1221–1232.

19. Schaffer, S. M., Tatini, S. R. and Bear, R. J., Microbiological safety of blue and cheddar cheese containing naturally modified milk fat. *J. Food Prot.*, 1995, 58, 132–138.

20. Subramanian, S., Transgenic therapeutics – medicines in milk. Biotechnology and Society–Part 22, 2004; www.chennaionline.com

21. Maga, E. A. and Anderson, G. B., The effect of mammary gland expression of human lysozyme on the properties of milk from transgenic mice. *J. Dairy Sci.*, 1995, 78, 2645–2652.

22. Lonnerdal, B., Recombinant human milk proteins – an opportunity and a challenge. *Am. J. Clin. Nutr.*, 1996, 63, 622S–626S.

23. Johnson, A. O., Semenya, J. G., Buchowski, M. S., Enwonwu, C. O. and Scrimshaw, N. S., Correlation of lactose maldigestion, lactose intolerance, and milk intolerance. *Am. J. Clin. Nutr.*, 1993, 57, 399–401.

24. Wal, J. M., Klaenhammer, T. R., Connolly, J. F., FitzGerald, R. J., Stanton, C. and Ross, R. P., Strategies for assessment and identification of allergenicity in (novel) foods. Special Issue: Functional foods: designer foods for the future, Cork, Irish Republic, 30 September–2 October 1997. *Int. Dairy J.*, 1998, 8, 413–423.

□□□

Chapter 14

Contract Farming as a Tool for Sustainable Development through Integration of Smallholder Livestock Farmers

AMANDEEP SINGH[1] AND PRANAV KUMAR[2]

[1] Research Scholar, Division of Extension Education, ICAR-Indian Veterinary Research Institute, Izatnagar, Bareilly, Uttar Pradesh, India (243122). E-mail : amandeepsinghvet@gmail.com

[2] Assistant Professor, Division of Veterinary & Animal Husbandry Extension Education, Faculty of Veterinary Sciences & Animal Husbandry, Sher-E-Kashmir University of Agricultural Sciences & Technology of Jammu, R.S. Pura, Jammu, Jammu & Kashmir, India (181102). E-mail : pranavahe@gmail.com

Introduction

The active and sustainable participation of smallholder livestock producers in the rapid growth and development of the livestock sector in the international arena is seen as bringing about a potential pathway for rural income growth and poverty alleviation in developing countries. However, the route by which these small holders can get truly involved and take advantage of opportunities in the growing livestock markets is not too clear as there exists a host of barriers to their participation that smallholders, on their own, find difficult to overcome. Over time, structural transformation in the agricultural sector of developing countries has seen the emergence and spread of contract farming in the production and marketing of agricultural products, in general and of livestock products in particular. The main objective of this article is to determine the extent to which contract farming and its variants enable smallholder livestock producers to gain market access, and explore other market institutions for more effectively integrating smallholders into the growth and development of the livestock sector in developing countries.

What is Contract Farming?

Contract Farming is essentially an agreement between unequal parties, companies, Government bodies or individual entrepreneurs on the one hand and economically weaker farmers on the other. The main feature of Contract Farming is that the buyer/contractor supplies all the material inputs and technical advice required for cultivation to the cultivator. This approach is widely used, not only for tree and cash crops but also, increasingly for fruits and vegetables, poultry, pigs, dairy products and even prawn and fish.

In a nutshell, contract farming is the businesses signing contracts with farmers to grow a specific crop, even a specific seed variety, and guaranteeing buy-back of the produce at an agreed price or price range, holds the promise that the next generation of yield improvements could come through efforts from the private sector.

History of Contract Farming in India

Contract farming can be traced back to colonial period when commodities like Collin Indigo were produced by the Indian farmers for English factories. Seed production has been carried out through contract farming by the seed companies quite successfully for more than four decades in the country. The new agricultural policy of 2000 sought to promote growth of private sector participation in agribusiness through contract farming and land bearing arrangements to accelerate technology transfers, capital inflows and assured market for crops.

The colonial period saw the introduction of cash crops such as tea, coffee, and rubber, poppy and indigo in various parts of the country, mostly through a central expatriate-owned estate surrounded by small out growers model. IndiaTobacco Company (ITC) introduced cultivation of Virginia tobacco in Coastal Andhra Pradesh in the 1920's incorporating most elements of a fair contract farming system and met with good farmer response. This was replaced by auctions in 1984. The Pepsico introduced tomato cultivation in Punjab in the 1990's under farming to obtain inputs for its paste-manufacturing facility established as a pre-condition to its entry in to India. This was sold to Hindustan Lever in 2000, which had earlier acquired the Kissan Karnataka. The PepsiCo's intervention and subsequent similar interventions by Hindustan Lever and Niger Agro Foods, are credited with transforming tomato cultivation in Punjab.Contract Farming was the strategy of choice for almost all food processing projects contemplated in the 1980's and 1990's.Until 2003, when reforms of the Agricultural Produce Market Committee Act was initiated in many states, it was illegal in most states for businesses to purchase agricultural produce directly from farmers rather than from government-regulated local markets called *mandis*.

Present Stage of Contract Farming in India

Today, contract farming is emerging as a preferred mechanism through which agri-businesses can directly engage with farmers. An expanding urban middle class and increasing commercial investment in agricultural retailing and processing are creating demand for more standardized, higher-quality agricultural produce. But under-developed supply chains and small farm sizes make sourcing such produce difficult.

The Union Agriculture Ministry is putting its weight behind contract farming drafting a model law to give legal support to a practice that can give small farmers access to modern technology and resources. The farm ministry detailed an agenda for expansion of agricultural credit to the tune of Rs.7, 36,570 crore during 10th five year Plan and the official note to the finance ministry gave financing of contract farming by banks priority. Agricultural and Processed Food Products Development Authority is developing policy guidelines on contract farming for forwarding to state governments for implementation. The guidelines will focus on regularizing the relation between producers and processors of food materials. During 10th five year plan, 20 Agri Export zones had set-up in different states that integrated the complete process from production to export stage and contract farming is being encouraged to rope in local farmers to join these export zones as members to pool in their produce.The National Agricultural Policy had highlighted the need for an increase in the private sector participation in farming by leasing private land for agri-business and contract farming to private companies. The Standing Committee on Food Management and Agricultural Exports had recommended suitable amendments to the State Agricultural Produce Marketing Regulation Act to promote development of marketing infrastructure in private and co-operative sectors, direct marketing and contract farming.

Contract farming is not totally new to our country. When the white revolution was born in India, contract farming also came into being by the introduction of Operation Flood Iand II. Milk cooperatives of Gujarat under the banner AMUL are running examples of a type of Contract farming. In livestock sector, contract farming is operating with success, especially in poultry farming and dairying. In case of poultry, there are some examples of successful contract farming like Suguna from Tamil Nadu. The contract poultry farming also carried out in state like Andhra Pradesh, Chhattisgarh, Haryana, Karnataka, Madhya Pradesh, Maharashtra, Punjab, Rajasthan, Uttrakhand, and Uttar Pradesh. In dairying there are some examples of successful contract farming like Nestle India's company in Punjab. The contract dairy farming also carried out in states like Andhra Pradesh, Chhattisgarh, Haryana, Karnataka, Madhya Pradesh, Maharashtra, Rajasthan, Uttrakhand, and Uttar Pradesh.

Types of Contract Farming

These are a few of the models of contract farming that are accepted globally:

- Centralized model
- Nucleus Estate model
- Multipartite model
- Informal model
- Intermediary model

Centralized Model

The contracting company provides support to the production of the crop by smallholder farmers, purchases the crop from the farmers, and then processes, packages and markets the product, thereby tightly controlling its quality. This can be used for crops such as tobacco, cotton, paprika, sugar cane, banana, coffee, tea, cocoa and rubber. This may involve tens of thousands of farmers. The level of involvement of the contracting company in supporting production may vary.

Nucleus Estate Model

This is a variation of the centralized model. The promoter also owns and manages an estate plantation (usually close to a processing plant) and the estate is often fairly large in order to provide some guarantee of throughput for the plant. It is mainly used for tree crops, but can also be for, e.g., fresh vegetables and fruits for export.

Multipartite Model

The multipartite model usually involves the government, statutory bodies and private companies jointly participating with the local farmers. The model may have separate organizations responsible for credit provision, production, management, processing and marketing of the produce.

Informal Model

This model is basically run by individual entrepreneurs or small companies who make simple, informal production contracts with farmers on a seasonal basis. The crops usually require only a minimal amount of processing or packaging for resale to the retail trade or local markets, as with vegetables, watermelons, and fruits. Financial investment is usually minimal. This is perhaps the most speculative of all contract-farming models, with a risk of default by both promoter and farmer.

Intermediary Model

This model has formal subcontracting by companies to intermediaries (collectors, farmer groups, NGOs) and the intermediaries have their own (informal) arrangements with farmers. The main disadvantage in this model is it disconnects the link between company and farmer.

Nature of Contracts in Contract Farming

In the investigation on the nature of contracts, their terms and conditions, the literature mainly deals with formal contracts. Adaptations of such modern formal contract agreements from industrialized countries are seen in the case countries of India, Thailand, Vietnam and the Philippines albeit these are modified according tothe institutional environment in the developing countries concerned. The nature of livestock production contracts engaged in by the integrator and the farmer differs according to the product in question in the transaction. Yet even for the same product, there are variations across countries that tend to be driven by the changing needs of the markets on certain product attributes, types of transaction costs that need to be hurdled, and the distribution of power between integrator and farmer.

Fixed-Fee or Wage Contracts

The integrator provides all intermediate inputs required to produce the output. The standard input-output ratios and quality attributes are stipulated. The farmer is then paid an agreed upon fee in exchange for his labour, management, and use of facilities. Under fixed-fee contracts, the integrator assumes the market risks of changes in input and output prices. The producer is insulated from risk, but does not share from the gains obtained from the realization of more favourable prices.

On the other hand, production risks impact on both parties when further complexities in the contract are introduced to include provisions for incentives and penalties based (FCR) and harvest recovery rate (HR) also work as a deterrent to producer 'cheating' (i.e., would mean lesser supervision and monitoring costs). The possible diversion of feeds and other inputs to other activities is a risk to the integrator, but agreed standards on FCR would mitigate the risks on the part of the integrator. Mortalities of livestock are also a risk to the integrator, but standard agreements on HR mitigate.

Forward-Price or Profit-Sharing Contracts

Forward-price and profit sharing contracts appear to be a mix of a market specification and management-providing contract, where the integrator ensures the marketing of the output, but is also involved in technical assistance at the farm production level in order to come up with the product characteristics demanded by the market. The degree of integrator involvement depends on the level of skills the farmer has acquired at the production level. These contracts, however, may also contain certain features of a resource-providing contract where the integrator assures the supply of the intermediate inputs but on credit at agreed-upon prices. The cost of these inputs is then charged to the farmer when the output is sold.

A minimum forward-price of output could be guaranteed to the producer. Where this guarantee is provided, the integrator assumes the market risk. Under profit-sharing contracts, in the case where the output price used to compute profits is the prevailing market price at the time of the disposal of output, the market risks are shared between the two, and so are the benefits to an output price increase. On the input prices side, the bearing of risks would depend on the treatment of input prices used. If at prevailing market prices, the risks are shared.

The production risk is either totally or partially borne by the producer, depending on the agreements pertaining to mortalities.

Formal Contracts

Formal contracts in broiler production are mainly of the fixed-fee type in India. In general, for formal contracts, when integrators are dealing with large or medium scale farmers, fixed-fee contracts are offered, and they exert quite a heavy market power relative to the producer, with as much production risk shifted to the producer. When producers have sufficient capacity to manage and control their production performance, and could undertake production independently by assuming all the market risks, guaranteed forward-price contracts emerge.

Informal Contracts

Informal contracts are more difficult to put into a box. Some have the characteristics of a simple resource providing contract in terms of the integrator assuring the supply of intermediate production inputs on credit, to be repaid when output is sold, but with no obligation on the part of the farmer to yield the output to the integrator for marketing the product. Some exhibit a combination of a management providing and resource providing contract, where the integrator extends technical services to obtain the volume and quality of product required. In general, informal contracts are mainly undertaken by small holders with market intermediaries in the interest of getting assured supply of intermediate inputs and live stock services on credit.

Why Contract Farming in India?

Contracts that provide credit, technology, inputs, information, extension services, and risk mitigation help producers to improve production efficiency; develop commercial culture and augment income and employment. Further contract farming is viewed as a tool to provide technology, extension service, and financial credit and assured market to the farmers. The proponents of contract farming view it is an avenue through which greater private sector participation in agriculture could be encouraged. In our country, the farmers face the problems of traditional technology and management practices, little bargaining power with input suppliers and produce markets, inadequate infrastructure and market information, lack of management expertise, poor package of produce and inadequate capital to grow a quality livestock. They are waiting for change for better living standards. Contract farming helps small farmers to purchase milch animals, increase production and benefit from market led growth. Contract farming will maximize the profits to the farmers and minimize risk in farming like production related risks, transfer price risk and produce risk. In informal contracts, there is generally a greater flexibility by market intermediaries in accommodating smallholder producers, as evidenced in dairy contracts in India.

Role of Contract Farming as an Extension Service

Although the public extension system in India is well-developed in terms of infrastructure and manpower, the delivery of services is inefficient. By adopting the contract farming many of extension services such as farm management and marketing through exchange of information among farmers, better use of existing technology, transfer of modern technology, building the farmers knowledge, capacities and skills, improvement in farmers living standards and feedback from field can be met easily.

Contract farming can act as solution to constraints of extension system, such as multiplicity of technology transfer systems because of lack of manpower, lack of farmer focus and feedback, inadequate technical capacity within the extension system, inadequate capacity building of farmers, present weak Research-Extension-Farmer-Market Linkages, inadequate operating resources and financial sustainability etc. Thus, the agricultural extension continues to be in transition and cherished dream Public Private Partnership (PPP) in transfer of technology can be made true easily. Stock of farm input supply and frequency of extension visits appeared to have negative influence. The study recommended follow-up visits coupled with quality extension services by extension agents after the introduction and adoption of new technology to farmers.

Advantages of contract farming for farmers

The prime advantage of a contractual agreement for farmers is that the sponsor will normally undertake to purchase all produce grown, within specified quality and quantity parameters. Contracts can also provide farmers with access to a wide range of managerial, technical andextension services that otherwise may be unobtainable.

Farmers can use the contract agreement as collateral to arrange credit with a commercial bank in order to fund inputs. Thus, the main potential advantages for farmers are:

1. Provision of inputs and production services.
2. Access to credit.
3. Introduction of appropriate technology.
4. Skill transfer.
5. Guaranteed and fixed pricing structures and.
6. Access to reliable markets.

Disadvantages of contract farming for farmers

For farmers, the potential disadvantages associated with contract farming include:

1. Increased risk.
2. Unsuitable technology and crop incompatibility.
3. Manipulation of quotas and quality specifications.
4. Corruption.
5. Domination by monopolies; and
6. Indebtedness and over reliance on advances.

Advantages of contract farming for sponsors

Companies and government agencies have a number of options to obtain raw materials for their processing and marketing activities. The benefits of contract farming are best examined in the light of the other alternatives, namely spot market purchases and large-scale estates. The main potential advantages for sponsors can be seen as:

1. Political acceptability.
2. Overcoming land constraints.
3. Production reliability and shared risk.
4. Quality consistency; and
5. Promotion of farm inputs.

Disadvantages of contract farming for sponsors

The main disadvantages faced by contract farming sponsors are:

1. Land availability constraints.
2. Social and cultural constraints.
3. Farmer discontent.
4. Extra-contractual marketing; and
5. Input diversion.

Contract Farming Ventures in India: A Few Successful Cases

1. **The Classic Case of Pepsi Foods Ltd. :** Launching its agro-business in India with special focus on exports of value-added processed foods, Pepsi Foods Ltd. ('PepsiCo'here after) entered India in 1989 by installing aRs 22 crorestate of-the-art tomato processing plant at Zahura in Hoshiarpur district of Punjab. The company intended to produce aseptically packedpastes and purees for the international market. However, before long, the company recognised that investment in agro-processing plants would not be viable unless the yields and quality of agricultural produce to be processed were up to international standards. At that point of time, tomato had never been cultivatedin Punjab for its solid content, with a focus on high yields andother desirable processing characteristics, such as colour, viscosity and water binding properties. The shortfall of tomatoes for running the factory led tothe birth of PepsiCo's backward linkage with farmers of Punjab.Pepsi Co. follows the contract farming method described earlier,where the grower plants the company's crops on his land, and the company provides selected inputs like seeds/ saplings, agricultural practices, and regular inspection of the crop and advisory serviceson crop management The Pepsi Co. model of contract farming, measured in terms of new options for farmers, productivity increases, and the introduction of modern technology, has been an unparalleled success.

2. **Appachi's Integrated Cotton Cultivation:Innovative Model :** Appachi Cotton Company (ACC), the ginning and trading house from Pollachi (Coimbatore district of Tamil Nadu, India) hit the head lines in May 2002 for the street play it employed to encourage farmers in the Nachipalayam village in

Kinathukadavu block of Coimbatore to sow cotton seeds in their fields. The singer in the street play assured cotton farmers that, unlike in the past, they would not be disappointed, if they cultivated cotton on their fields,as they would be backed by a model called the Integrated Cotton Cultivation (ICC), which would guarantee a market-supportive mechanism for selling their produce.

The Appachi formula ensured that its farmer members never went short of money and materials during the crucial 100 days of the crop cycle. The contract assured the farmers easy availability of quality seeds, farm finance at an interest rate of 12% per annum,door delivery of unadulterated fertilisers and pesticides at discounterates, expert advice and field supervision every alternate week, anda unique selling option through a MoU with the co-ordinating agency (ACC). The core principle of the formula lies in the formation of farmers'Self-Help Groups (SHGs).

3. **Ugar Sugar's Experience With Barley :** The story of the Belgaum (Karnataka) based Ugar Sugar Work Ltd., which established a successful backward linkage with farmersof Northern Karnataka for supply of barley for its malt unit, is quite interesting and insightful. Farmers surrounding Ugar Sugarin Belgaum, who had been cultivating sugar under intens iveirrigation found themselves with the problem of salinity in soils.Ugar Sugar took this opportunity to begin creating awareness amongthe farming community about alternative crops suitable for saline soils. of these, barley was known to give economic yields of good quality in saline soils. The company assured the farmers of a markefor their produce, if they agreed to grow barley, as well as the required technical and input support.All this happened way back in 1997, when the company required 5000 tons of barley annually for its malt unit. At that point oftime, barley was cultivated on a commercial scale only in thenorthern parts of India, which meant huge transportation costs forthe company to source from there. Further more, such lots carried amixture of feed and malt grade barley, which meant no surety of consistent quality raw material. The company had no land of itsown to start barley production near its malt plant. This led to the birth of Ugar Sugar's unique contract farming system for barley production.

4. **Poultry Venture by Suguna :** With the presence in more than 16 states in India, Suguna foods have integrated more than 23,000 poultry farmers in India with a vision to "Energize Rural India". Suguna under contract farming model provide farmers with measures to optimize production. Company owned feed mills, research and development centres, processing plants, training programmes, hatcheries, technology infrastructure are used by the farmers in contract with the company.

5. **Nestle Progressing in Dairy Contracts :** Nestle focuses on the technical assistance, financial assistance, promotion of husbandry practices and farming training and education. With all the provisions, today Nestle works with around 11,000 dairy farmers and collects more than 300 million kilograms of milk every year across Punjab, Haryana and Rajasthan.

Conclusion

Contract Farming is not a panacea to solve all related problems of agricultural production and marketing systems. But contract farming could be evaluated as a way of providing earlier access to credit, input, information and technology and product markets for the small scale farming structure. Contract farming might also be seen as a way or as a part of rural development and promoted to improve agricultural performance, especially in Third World Countries.

There is an urgent need to integrate the small and marginal farmers so that the resources can be pooled for common interests and more productivity can be reached. Integration will not only enhance the production but will also stop the migration of the rural youth towards urban areas in search of job. It also promises better adoption and diffusion of technologies by the farmers thereby enhancing their skills too. Contract farming also promises the easy marketing of the produce from the door steps of the farmers thereby reducing worries related to marketing of the produce, which is one of the major constraints faced by the rural farmers. On the whole, contract farming has many prospects when it comes to boosting the rural economy and hence, it can be projected and advocated as prosperous system of livestock farming among the rural livestock farmers.

References

Angeles, M., Catelo, O. and Costales, A.C. (2008).Contract Farming and Other Market Institutions as Mechanisms for Integrating Smallholder Livestock Producers in the Growth and Development of the Livestock Sector in Developing Countries.PPLPI Working Paper 45.

Eaton, C. and Shepherd, A.W. (2001).Contract Farming: Partnerships for growth.FAO Agricultural Services Bulletin, Rome.ISBN 92-5-104593-3 (pp.41-56).

Gulati, A., Joshi, P.K. and Landes, M (2008). Contract Farming in India : A Resource Book. A Product of Indo-US Knowledge Initiative on Agriculture jointly published by ICAR, IFPRI and USDA.

Kolekar, D.V., Kokate, L.S., Bangar, Y.C. and Khillare, G.S. (2012). Review on contract dairy farming : to boost Indian dairying. Livestock Research for rRural Development : Volume 24; article 181.

Kumar, A. (2011). India Journal : The Rise of Contract Farming. Wall Street Journal: Jul 20, 2011.

Shoja Rani, B. N. (2007). Globalization and Contract Farming in India-Advantages and Problems.*Conference on Global Competition & Competitiveness of Indian Corporate.Retrieved from www.dspace.iimk.ac.in/handle/2259/51.*

Spice (2003). Vol. 1 No. 4 : March 2003. Spice is a bi-monthly publication from The National Institute of Agricultural Extension Management (MANAGE), an organisation of the Ministry of Agriculture, Govt. of India.

❑❑❑

Chapter 15

Sources of Communication for Farming Community in India

Y.S. BAGAL[1], L.K. SHARMA[2] AND PRANAV KUMAR[3]

[1] Research Scholar, Division of Agricultural Extension Education, FoA, SKUAST-Jammu

[2] Associate Professor, Division of Agricultural Extension Education, FoA, SKUAST-Jammu

[3] Assistant Professor, Division of Veterinary & Animal Husbandry Extension Education, Faculty of Veterinary Sciences & Animal Husbandry, SKUAST-Jammu

---

Information on agriculture, both crop and livestock was communicated among farmers from ancient times. However, with the development in agricultural and livestock research, the need arises to rapidly and accurately transfer new information and technologies to the end user i.e. farmers. To fulfill this need media (print and electronic) and interpersonal communication has proved its usefulness in creating awareness about new agricultural technologies. As All India Radio played a significant role during the era of green revolution by disseminating the information regarding high yield varieties. Along with high yielding seeds and irrigation facilities, the enthusiasm of farmers mobilized the idea of the agricultural revolution and is also credited to All India Radio. The success of agricultural development programmes largely depends on the nature and extent of use of communication sources. A study conducted by Kapoor (2015) found that radio (97.5%), television (86.25%), fellow farmers (71.25%), newspaper (26.25%) and magazine (5%) were utilized by the respondents.

Interpersonal sources such as personal localite and personal cosmopolite comprises of like extension agents, friends, family members, fellow farmers, neighbours, group discussions, demonstrations, campaign and village leaders, etc. These sources play a significant role in dissemination of information related to agriculture. During the pre-independence era, interpersonal communication channels were used widely as in Sriniketan and Marthandam projects. Demonstration centers were established to disseminate information by conducted demonstration under the guidance of experts. Before independence, nationwide programme was launched in mid of 1940s, to overcome the effect of Bengal famine, and campaign method was used namely "Grow More Food Campaign". It focused on the dissemination of the technical information related to agriculture through posters and slogans. As per Kumawat, *et al.* (2014) who conducted a study entitled, "Knowledge and information source utilization pattern of arid legume growers in Jalore district of Rajasthan" revealed that among personal cosmopolite sources, the credibility of KVK scientists, agriculture supervisors and Assistant Agricultural Officers was found higher as compared to other cosmopolite sources. In case of personal localite sources, fellow farmers and telephones/ mobile were having maximum credible score. They further revealed that radio and leaflet had maximum credibility in case of impersonal cosmopolite sources. Bhagat, *et al.* (2004) in a study on information sources for agricultural technology conducted in Jammu district on J&K state found that contact farmers were consulted by the respondents to the greatest extent in receiving information regarding agriculture, followed by extension personnel of Department of Agriculture, television, radio, scientists of agricultural university, farm magazines, newspapers and agricultural films (in decreasing order).

Mass media (print and electronic) were also used to disseminate information in its various capacities and formats. Mass media are those channels of communication, which reach to a large numbers of people at the same time and provide same information. They include media which spread information by sound (radio, audio cassettes); moving pictures (television, film, video); and print (posters, newspapers, leaflets). In a country like India, where literacy level is low, the choice of communication media is of vital importance. In this regard the television and radio are significant, as they transfer modern agricultural technology to literate and illiterate farmers alike even in interior areas, within short time. In India, farm and home broadcast with agricultural thrust were introduced in 1966, to enlighten farmers on the use of various technologies to boost agricultural development. The attraction of mass media to extension services is its high speed and low cost with which information can be communicated to people. Although the cost of producing and transmitting a radio programme may seem high, when that cost is divided between the millions of people who may hear the programme, it is in fact a very cheap way of providing information. Kardak, et al. (2004) reported that this respondents used to obtain information through contact with Friends (67.33%), proprietor of agro service center (56%) progressive farmers (55.33%), participation in Shivapheri (50%) and Shetkari Melawa (48.67%), hearing farm radio broadcast (66.67%) and watching of farm TV telecast (47.33%) sometimes. However, majority of the respondents were found to be not making use of Sarpanch, garmsevak, extension workers of Panchayat Samiti, magazine/farm literature and Krishi diary/Dainandini.

Among the several mass media, newspaper and farm magazine is commonly used. They have a vital role to play in the communication of agricultural information among the literate farmers. The print media widened the scope of communication. It is cheap and people can afford to buy and read them at their convenience. Newspaper, pamphlets, magazines, newsletters, leaflets, banners, wall-paintings, books/ booklets, brochures etc. not only disseminate accurate information to the farmers but also helps in preserving this information. Farm publications had proved to be effective means for dissemination of information, especially to introduce new technologies and are useful for disseminating information among literate farmers (Singh, 2001). For speedy transfer of agricultural technologies to the farmers, the Ministry of Agriculture and Farmers Welfare and Department of Agriculture and Cooperation started the scheme 'Use of Print Media in Technology Transfer' is being implemented through 31 State Agricultural Universities by contracting 2-3 major daily newspapers to bring out regular weekly/fortnightly columns on current agricultural news and practices in regional languages. Abbas et al., (2003) in their study in the central Punjab concluded that majority of the farmers consulted pamphlets, magazines, and newspapers for getting the information regarding sugarcane production technologies.

According to Ani, *et al.* (2015) who conducted a study on utilization of mass media among farmers in Ik were local government area of rivers state, Nigeria found that television (90.83%) was the most available mass media in the study area followed by radio (89.17%), mobile phone (81%), pamphlets/handbills (79.17%), posters (75%) and bulletins/newspapers/magazine (72.50%). However, computer and internet (37.5%) and e- mail (14.17%) were least available mass media in the study area.

Similarly, Devaraj and Ravichandran (2014) in a study on the role of information and mass media communication technology among farming community of Mandya District, Karnataka found that 36 percent of the respondents had high level of awareness about farm broadcast followed by moderate (34.75 per cent) and low level of awareness (29.25 per cent). Regarding farm telecasts (35.75 percent) of the respondents had high level of awareness followed by moderate (32.88 per cent) and low levels (31.05 per cent). The awareness level of the respondents regarding the farm programmes appear in radio and television could be moderate (33.81 per cent) followed by low (30.37 per cent) and high (35.81 per cent).

Indian Farming, Kheti, Phal Phool, Krishika and Modern Kheti are some of the popular Indian farm magazines, which have a very large circulation among its subscribers. Newspaper can support extension by publishing news of various extension activities, guidance and recommendations, achievements, market news, research findings, successful achievements and problems faced by farming community.

Apart from print-media, electronic media in the form of radio, television (T.V), internet, mobile phones, recordings (CD's, DVD's etc.) has also made significant contributions to the transfer of technologies. Those farmers who cannot effectively read the printed material can get the desired information through their electronic medium of communication.

Radio is a popular medium for infotainment as well as attitude change (Ray, 2003). Radio from its very inception played an important role in development communication. The international organizations like United Nations Children's Fund (UNICEF), United Nations Educational Scientific Cultural Organization (UNESCO) and Food and Agricultural Organization (FAO) have been using radio for the development in respective fields since 1960. (Chapman, R. *et. al*, 2003). It plays a peculiar role in technology dissemination (Ejembi *et al.*, 2006; Prathap and Ponnusamy, 2006). It is very effective media, which can reach effectively to the rural people. All India Radio has been the forerunner in the process of implementing communication strategy adopted by the government. Mass Media Support 100 Broadcast Sector to Agriculture Extension with the title Kisan Vani for AIR from 15th February, 2004 in collaboration with the Ministry of Agriculture to inform local farmers the daily market rates, weather reports and day-to-day activities in their area at micro level. The Radio Rural Form experiment of 1956, covered 156 villages and contained 30 minutes duration program twice a week on different issues like agriculture and varied subjects. (Choudhary, 2011) Radio programmes like Utam Khetti, Kisan Vani, Navi Chetana are disseminating the agriculture related information to the farmers in J&K.

Television is an ideal medium to convey information and news to illiterate and literate, urban and rural viewers on whom it would have profound impact (Lal, 2012). For such reason, television is used in a planned manner to motivate people to participate in developmental programs. T.V in India was introduced in 1959, on an experimental basis. In 1967, Delhi Television centre launched Krishi Darshan Program at the behest of Dr. Bikram Sarabhai and Prof. R. S. Swaminathan. The objective of this program was popularization of modern method in agriculture through television. (Choudhury, 2011). Kheda Communication Project was launched in 1975-89, under this 607 community television sets have been installed in 443 villages of Kheda district of Gujarat. The programmes mainly concentrate on the problems of poorer classes. T.V programmes like Nav Krishi, Krishi Darshan have gained popularity as they have been able to solve numerous ground level problems of the farmers and also replaced their antiquated technique with new innovations.

A study on impact of mass media on farmers agricultural production, case study of Borno state, agricultural development programme found that radio is most effective, followed by telephone calls and meeting with colleague and local leaders. The variables considered under each method include; face to face contact methods (16%), telephone calls (35%), letters and correspondence (14%). Also under the groups contact method, meetings (98%) field trips and excursions (9%), exhibition (6%); and demonstrations (19%). Mass methods are radio (96%), television (14%) and newspapers (10%). Others are printed materials (21%). (Shuwa, *et al.*, 2015).

Extension can reach more clients through mobile-based learning platforms- textual or richer platforms, such as video that provide tips to the farmers to improve agricultural skills and knowledge. Kisan Call Centres with toll free dial of 1800 180 1551 has provided the farmers an advantage to talk in their local language and getting advices from experts with the help of mobile. Many other initiatives like IFFCO Kisan Samachar Ltd., Mandi on Mobile, Reuters Market Light communicate information directly to farmers through mobiles. Internet plays a vital role in exchange of information through e-mails etc. Computers started in the Indian Society around 1986. The actual transition in India happened after 1996.

Conclusion

Communication plays a vital role in all social changes. Studies in India and global have pointed out that there is need for an effective communication to enable new innovations as well as research results to reach the farmers fields without much time lag. There is need for rapidly change from traditional to modern ways of life essentially involves communication of new ideas and their unhesitating acceptance by people. For this purpose, various communication media ranging from the sophisticated TV to the common and causal ones like interpersonal channels to modern ICT tools have to be utilized. Adoption of improved practices by the farmers varies from one farmer to farmer depending upon their situation and availability of information sources. Individuals tend to use different communication sources and channels for obtaining technology. There is a need to know more about favoured information sources and channels of farmers which would enable effective transfer of technologies.

References

Abbas, M., Sheikh, A.D., Muhammad, S. and Ashfaq, M. 2003. Role of print media in the dissemination of recommended sugarcane production technologies among farmers in the central Punjab- Pakistan. *International Journal of Agricultural Biological*, **5**: 26-9.

Ani, A.O., Umunakwe, P.C., Ejiogu-Okereke, E.N., Nwakwasi, R.N. and Aja, A.O. 2015. Utilization of Mass Media among Farmers in Lk were Local Government Area of Rivers State, Nigeria. *IOSR Journal of Agriculture and Veterinary Science*, **8**(1): 41-47.

Bhagat, G.R., Nain, M.S. and Nanda, Rakesh. 2004. Information sources for agricultural technology. *Indian Journal of Extension Education*, **40**(1 & 2): 111-112.

Chapman, Robert., Blench, Roger., Kranjac-Berisavljevic, Gordana. and Zakariah, A.B.T. 2003. Rural radio in agricultural extension: the example of vernacular radio programmes on soil and water conservation in N. Ghana. *Agriculture Research and Extension Network*, Network paper no. 127.

Choudhury, Payel Sen. 2011. Media in developmental communication. *Global Media Journal- Indian Edition*, **2**(2).

Devaraj and Ravichandran,P. 2014. A study on the role of information and mass media communication technology among farming community of Mandya District, Karnataka State, *Journal of Advances in Library and Information Science*, **3**(1): 43-46.

Ejembi, E.P., Omoregbee, F.E. and Ejembi, S.A. 2006. Farmers' assessment of the training and visit extension system in central Nigeria: evidence from Barkin Ladi, plateau state. *Journal Social Science*, **12**(3): 207-212.

Kardak, V.N., Kashid, N.V., Kamble, M.S. and Kardak, S.N. 2004. The socio-economic, communication and psychological characteristics of the sorghum growers in Vidharbha region in Maharashtra. *Annals of Agricultural Research*, **25**(2): 292-296.

Kumawat, S.R. and Singh, P. 2014. Knowledge and information source utilization pattern of arid legume growers. *Journal of Food Legumes*, **27**(1): 56-59.

Lal, Banarsi. 2012. Association between Attitude of Respondents towards Farm T.V. Programmes and Selected Independent Variable in Jammu and Kashmir, India. *Journal of Communication*, **3**(1): 47-49.

Pratap, D.P. and Ponnusamy, K.A. 2006. Mass media and symbolic adoption behaviour of rural women. Stud. Media Inform. Literacy Educ, **6**(4): 1-6.

Ray, G.L. 2003. *Extension Communication and Management*. (5th ed. Rev.) Kalyani Publisher, New Delhi, India.

Shuwa, M.I., Shettima, L., Makinta, B.G. 2015. Impact of mass media on farmers agricultural production, case study of Borno state, agricultural development programme. *Academic Journal of Scientific Research*, **3**(1): 008-014.

Singh, A.K., 2001. *Agricultural Extension: Impact and Assessment*. Agrobios, Jodhpur, India.

□□□

Chapter 16

Current Status of the Financial Inclusion of Livestock Farmers into Formal Economy of India

AMANDEEP SINGH[1] AND PRANAV KUMAR[2]

[1] Research Scholar, Division of Extension Education, ICAR-Indian Veterinary Research Institute,Izatnagar, Bareilly, Uttar Pradesh, India (243122). E-mail: amandeepsinghvet@gmail.com

[2] Assistant Professor, Division of Veterinary & Animal Husbandry Extension Education, Faculty of Veterinary Sciences & Animal Husbandry, Sher-E-Kashmir University of Agricultural Sciences & Technology of Jammu, R.S. Pura, Jammu, Jammu & Kashmir, India (181102). E-mail: pranavahe@gmail.com

India is an agricultural economy with more than 65 per cent population practicing agriculture and deriving livelihoods out of it. The contribution of agriculture to national GDP has crossed 27 per cent in the previous financial year. The contribution of livestock to national GDP is 4.11 per cent with almost 30 per cent workforce involved in livestock farming. Out of this huge manpower of 38 crores practicing animal husbandry, only 10 per cent livestock farmers above poverty line are associated with formal sources of livestock credit, remaining depends on informal sources for loaning their enterprises. Talking about the formal and informal sources of finance, the formal sources includes the banks and the co-operatives which follow the guidelines of the Reserve Bank of India and informal sources are those which include borrowing loans from NGOs, friends, local money lenders and relatives, etc. The striking difference between the two is the increased amount of interest rate and no collateral against finance in case of informal sources. The money borrowed and interest paid along with other transactions in case of informal finance remains out of the national exchequer and does not taken into account into the indicators of national development. In India about 86 per cent of the monetary transactions related to agriculture and allied sectors take place through informal channel of the economy which ultimately leads to exploitation of the farmers and undue advantage is taken by the money lenders.

According to ILO India Labour Market Update (2016) and NSSO data (2011-12), more than 90 per cent of the employment in the agricultural sector and close to 70 per cent in the non-agricultural sector falls under the informal category.Clearly, the informal sector is not the residual sector of the economy. In reality, it is the dominant sector. At present, only 10% of India's over 470 million workforces are in the formal sector. In other words, 90% of India's workers do not have the privileges—like social security and workplace benefits—enjoyed by their counter parts who are formally employed. It is estimated by NSSO that 84.7% of jobs in the Indian economy are in the informal or unorganized sector. Of this, excluding agriculture, the leading contributors of informal employment are manufacturing, construction and trade. Informal workers also work under worse working conditions with little job security, no perks or protections and with low wages. The protections guaranteed to workers under different legislations are not complied with by the informal sector, and they also escape the purview of the authorities. A large informal sector also impacts the government in terms of revenue foregone because units operating in the informal sector stay out of the government's fiscal revenue net (This leads to low tax GDP ratio). Hence, the informal sector is detrimental to the interests of the working population, the government and in the long run, even to the employer.

The government had started Pradhan Mantri Jan DhanYojana, Atal Pension Yojana, Pradhan Mantri Mudra Yojana with the establishment of MUDRA Bank, etc. for the financial inclusion of the informal institutions in general and the workers in particular but the results of the same seems to be undetermined. Pradhan Mantri Jan DhanYojana was launched with great success as more than 5.64 crores of bank accounts were opened for the financial inclusion of poor. As far as the financial inclusion of the livestock farmers is concerned, no such data is available but sources reveal that most of the live stock farmers are under the informal economy. The lives tock farmers borrow money from the money lenders, input dealers; procure feed, medicine, equipments from input dealers on credit, which levy high interest rates on the purchase. Further, the livestock farmers obtain informal credit from the NGOs and other producer companies. The producer companies like feed manufacturing companies, equipment manufacturing companies, product processing companies, etc. work with the farmers in integration and lift their produce for self-utilization and pay very low remuneration for the same. Some companies trap farmers into some contract whereby they provide farmers with initial seed money to start the farming and then enslave him for rest of the duration of farming which makes farmer to incur loss. Livestock farmers also borrow money from the money lenders, friends, etc. on high interest rates for purchasing new animals, for treatment of their sick animals, for purchasing feed, equipments, and remain in debted for long periods.

As far as the formal economy is concerned, only 10 per cent of the farmers procure loans from the banks and co-operatives in India. The apex institution for rural credit services in India i.e. National Bank for Agricultural and Rural Development (NABARD) works with Ministry of Agriculture, Government of India for dispensing loans to the farmers under various schemes launched by the government time to time.The project report for sanctioning of credit for the farmer is made by the Regional Rural Banks (RRBs) or Commercial Banks of the region and is sent to NABARD for sanctioning. The NABARD sanction the loan amount to the concerned bank, which further dispense the amount to the concerned farmer in phases of setting up of project and production of the commodity. All the livestock development schemes under National Livestock Mission (NLM) are liable for loan and livestock farmers can approach their local banks for making project report and sanctioning of funds.

Now-a-days, the microfinance institutions are increasing day by day which are providing credit services to the rural population and also developing their skills. The microfinance institutes are Self-Help Groups, Non-Governmental Organizations, which are registered by the government. There are some commercial banks like ICICI, HDFC ,which has started their own microfinance divisions in the rural areas for providing rural credit for farming as well as for purchasing house hold entities. Over the last ten years, however, successful experiences in providing finance to small entrepreneur and producers demonstrate that poor people, when given access to responsive and timely financial services at market rates, repay their loans and use the proceeds to increase their income and assets. This is not surprising since the only realistic alternative for them is to borrow from informal market at an interest much higher than market rates. Community banks, NGOs and grassroot savings and credit groups around the world have shown